Tips *for*
GOOD LIVING
with Arthritis

Editorial Director: Bethany Afshar
Art Director: Susan Siracusa
Illustrations: Jeffrey Pelo

Table *of* Contents

Acknowledgments

The Arthritis Foundation's *Tips for Good Living with Arthritis* is written for people who have one of the more than 100 forms of arthritis and arthritis-related diseases. Bringing this book to completion was a team effort, including the significant contributions of dedicated physicians, health-care professionals, Arthritis Foundation volunteers, writers, editors, designers and Arthritis Foundation staff.

Special acknowledgments should go to Susan Bernstein, who wrote the text, Susan Siracusa, who designed the cover and interior, and Jeffrey Pelo, the artist who created the illustrations.

The chief medical reviewer of the book is John H. Klippel, MD, the President and CEO of the Arthritis Foundation. This book was also medically reviewed by Leena Sharma, MD, Professor of Medicine, Rheumatology Department, Northwestern University, Evanston, IL; Patricia Grosklaus, PT, of Dunwoody, GA; and Pamela Harrell, OT, Arthritis and Osteoporosis Care Center, Nashville, TN.

Introduction

When you have arthritis – and more than 66 million Americans do have some arthritis-related condition at the dawn of the 21st century – daily life can be filled with many challenges, both physical and mental. Ordinary activities you once took for granted, from driving to climbing stairs to doing laundry, can be difficult and painful when you have arthritis. You may feel stressed, depressed, tired and angry at your pain and loss of independence.

You don't have to let the stiffness, pain, swelling and fatigue associated with arthritis keep you from doing what you need and love to do. You *can* take control of your arthritis and achieve good living.

By following the joint protection tips explained in this book, you can become a successful *self-manager* – a person who takes steps to overcome the symptoms of arthritis and live a full life. Self-management includes following a good diet, exercising regularly, avoiding unhealthy habits and using new techniques and assistive devices to help perform daily activities with arthritis.

Tips for Good Living With Arthritis is your guide to achieving a healthier, more productive life with arthritis.

There are many other resources of help and information for you, including the Arthritis Foundation's programs, services, interactive Web site and publications. There are more than 100 Arthritis Foundation chapters and offices all around the country. To find a chapter near you, call **800/283-7800** or visit to the Arthritis Foundation Web site at **www.arthritis.org**.

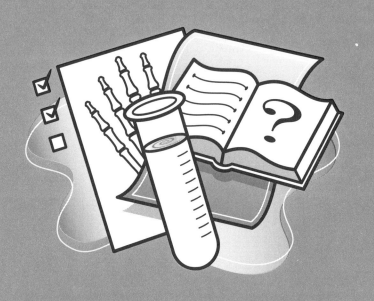

MORE THAN ACHES AND PAINS:
What *is* Arthritis?

Arthritis is a term that describes not just one disease but more than 100 different conditions. Arthritis – a combination of the Greek words *arth* (joint) and *itis* (inflammation) – means joint inflammation. When a person has arthritis, joints and surrounding tissues, such as muscles or tendons, often become inflamed. Inflammation is the body's reaction to illness or injury, which can cause pain, swelling, redness or heat in certain areas, such as a joint.

Arthritis and related diseases are also known as *rheumatic diseases*. This term describes diseases of the joints, muscles and connective tissues, each having different causes. There are some very serious forms of arthritis that are called *autoimmune* diseases. In these diseases, the body's *immune system* malfunctions. The immune system is a term that refers to the body's network of defenses against such disease-causing agents as viruses or bacteria. In forms of arthritis that are autoimmune diseases, such as rheumatoid arthritis, the body's disease-fighting components mistakenly turn against the body itself, causing damage to joints, cartilage, skin and other organs.

Most forms of arthritis are *chronic* diseases, which means they will be with you for the rest of your life. They do not go away and cannot, at this time, be "cured" by a drug or treatment. Chronic diseases differ from *acute* diseases, such as pneumonia or the flu, which are resolved on their own or are cured by drugs.

Just because arthritis is chronic doesn't mean that a person with the disease constantly experiences such symptoms as pain or inflammation. Arthritis symptoms have periods of *flare*, when symptoms are active, and *remission*, when symptoms subside.

Similarly, having arthritis doesn't mean you can't enjoy a full, active lifestyle. You can experience life fully with the help of treatments prescribed by your physician and steps outlined in this book that will help you take control of your arthritis and protect your joints from further damage.

There is no known cure for arthritis, and in many cases, no certain cause for why the disease develops. However, new research is shedding light on why arthritis may develop, what actions may prevent some forms of the disease, and what medical treatments and lifestyle changes delay or halt further, debilitating joint damage.

What happens when you have arthritis?

Arthritis is not a single disease, as many people believe. Arthritis is a complex collection of many different diseases with varied symptoms. Pain is one common thread between the more than 100 different arthritis-related conditions. Arthritis usually involves pain in or around the joints, although the intensity of this pain varies from person to person.

Arthritis also may cause inflammation, or swelling, in and around the joint. Other common symptoms are stiffness and limited mobility. As a result of arthritis pain and inflammation, people also may experience fatigue and sleeplessness, or even depression. There are effective treatments available for all of these symptoms.

Each form of arthritis or arthritis-related condition has its own symptoms and set of criteria for diagnosis. In addition, they each have their own treatments that your physician will prescribe or advise you to follow. Based on a physical examination, which may include lab tests, measures of physical function and a thorough discussion of your symptoms, your physician will diagnose your disease and begin to develop a treatment plan with you. Many arthritis symptoms develop gradually, so it may take time before you recognize the problem and get an accurate diagnosis from your physician. Be patient and persistent in order to find the proper diagnosis and path of treatment.

You can take control of arthritis symptoms by making positive changes in your lifestyle. Losing excess pounds if you are overweight can reduce stress to your joints, particularly the hip or knee. Regular, sensible exercise can strengthen muscles that support damaged joints. You may wish to refrain from drinking alcohol, which may increase the risk of side effects from drugs used to treat arthritis. Excess alcohol use also may cause your overall health to decline. You can learn new ways to perform daily activities that protect your joints and may reduce further damage, pain and swelling.

Incorporating the right lifestyle habits is key to good living with arthritis, and this book will give you tips on how to do just that.

COMMON ARTHRITIS MYTHS

Although arthritis has been around for thousands of years – anthropologists found evidence of the disease in excavated Ice Age skeletons –

most people still misunderstand this disease. Here, we will try to reveal the truth behind the most common myths about arthritis.

Myth: *Arthritis is just another term for the aches and pains you get as you grow older.*

Arthritis is more prevalent as people age, but arthritis can develop at any age. Very young children get arthritis, and some elderly people never develop the disease. Arthritis is a complex disease that can cause serious pain and joint damage. Although some forms of arthritis or other musculoskeletal conditions may stay stable without specific medical treatment, other forms, such as rheumatoid arthritis, may be debilitating.

Myth: *Arthritis is not a serious health problem.*

The various forms of arthritis and rheumatic diseases, taken as a whole, comprise the most common chronic health condition in the United States. Arthritis and related conditions affect about one in every six people. In the older population, arthritis and related diseases are even more common, and this population is swelling due to the aging of the post-World War II, baby-boom generation.

Arthritis is the leading cause of disability. For example, less than half of rheumatoid arthritis patients younger than 65 who are working when the disease develops are able to do their jobs 10 years later.

The impact of arthritis on the American economy is huge. By some estimates, costs associated with arthritis amount to $128 billion a year. These costs fall into three categories: direct, indirect and intangible. *Direct* medical costs include fees for physicians and other health-care professionals, as well as costs of laboratory tests and X-rays, drugs, assistive devices, surgeries and other treatments. There also are *indirect* costs. People with arthritis may lose their work income when they have to quit their job or make arrangements to go on disability leave. Finally, arthritis entails *intangible* costs, such as travel expenses for medical care or costs incurred when a spouse must take medical leave from his or her job to care for the person with arthritis.

Myth: *You can't do much about the pain and disability associated with arthritis.*

Currently, there is no cure for arthritis or other rheumatic conditions. However, that doesn't mean arthritis pain, inflammation, stiffness and other symptoms cannot be treated effectively. There are many over-the-counter medications and topical creams that can relieve minor arthritis pain and inflammation. For more severe symptoms, your physician can prescribe a number of drugs to relieve the symptoms of arthritis and prevent damage to your joints. In addition, you can try simple, nondrug techniques to combat arthritis symptoms. These methods include treating a painful joint with a heating pad or trying new exercises to keep joints loose.

There are many medications used to treat the symptoms of arthritis. These treatments include *nonsteroidal anti-inflammatory drugs* (NSAIDs), such as aspirin or ibuprofen; *corticosteroids*, such as prednisone; and *disease-modifying antirheumatic drugs* (DMARDs), such as methotrexate. In addition, many people with arthritis take *analgesics*, such as acetaminophen, to fight pain.

Arthritis research yields new medical treatments all the time. Due to recent breakthroughs, there are drugs called *COX-2 inhibitors* that treat inflammation without causing the stomach distress associated with traditional NSAIDs. For treating people with serious forms of inflammatory arthritis, such as rheumatoid arthritis, there is a class of drugs called *biologic response modifiers* (BRMs). These drugs block chemicals in the body that cause inflammation and joint damage.

Furthermore, damaged joints may be repaired through various surgical treatments or replaced with man-made joints. For most people with arthritis, a very effective way of controlling pain and stiffness is by adopting joint-protection techniques and healthy lifestyle changes, a practice known as *self-management*.

In addition to practicing self-management, it is important for all people with arthritis to have a comfortable partnership with their physicians and the other health professionals who assist them in managing their disease.

SUCCESS THROUGH SELF-MANAGEMENT

If you don't have a healthy lifestyle or change certain unhealthy habits, arthritis can escalate and lead to disability. A generation ago, most people assumed that this course was inevitable. That assumption isn't true, but you must take an active role in self-managing your lifestyle and daily activities.

Successful self-managers of arthritis are people who seize control of their own care. They engage their physicians in interactive dialogue about their care. They adopt good-living strategies, including a healthy diet, regular exercise and stretching. They actively protect their joints from damage, whether by modifying their activities or adapting their home and work surroundings with *assistive devices* – products designed to help the person with arthritis do various daily tasks.

No matter what form of arthritis you have, or what level of joint damage you experience, self-management is the cornerstone to battling pain, stiffness and immobility. Taking control of your care and being a successful self-manager are the keys to good living with arthritis.

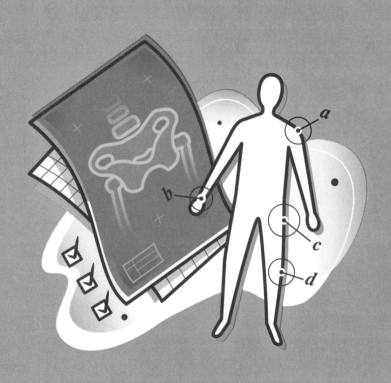

ARTHRITIS:
Many Different Diseases

As we learned in the first chapter, arthritis isn't just one disease, but a collective term describing more than 100 different diseases and related conditions. Common symptoms of these diseases include pain and inflammation. However, these diseases affect people in different ways, have different possible causes and are treated with different medications and self-management techniques.

For all forms of arthritis, there are ways to help manage pain and other symptoms. It's important for anyone with arthritis to develop good living habits. These habits include adopting a low-fat, healthy diet to keep weight under control, and incorporating an exercise routine to keep bodies fit and joints loose.

Osteoarthritis

The most common form of arthritis is *osteoarthritis*. Osteoarthritis also is known as OA, degenerative joint disease or osteoarthrosis. Osteoarthritis affects more than 27 million Americans. It usually develops gradually after age 40. Before age 45, the disease is more common in men. After 45, OA is more prevalent in women.

Most people associate osteoarthritis with aging or with older people. In fact, young people also can develop osteoarthritis, especially people who may damage their joints through injury or repetitious use. Some athletes or people who do physical labor develop osteoarthritis as a result of injury to joints. Years of wear and tear on joints can lead to osteoarthritis in older people, but other factors help determine whether or not you develop the condition.

Osteoarthritis results from the breakdown of *cartilage* in the joints, leading to pain and stiffness. Cartilage is the smooth, rubbery substance that covers the ends of bones, acting as a cushion between bones that come together to form a joint. Cartilage allows the bones to move properly and prevents bone-on-bone contact. When cartilage breaks down, the ends of bones may rub together, causing pain, stiffness and decreased mobility.

Osteoarthritis occurs most frequently in the joints of the neck, knees, hands, fingers, hips and spine. Usually, OA does not affect the same joint on both sides of the body – one knee, for example, instead of both knees. However, some people do develop OA in the same joint on both sides of the body.

As you age, cartilage may wear thin or change, losing its elasticity and becoming more easily damaged. When the cartilage breaks down, as in osteoarthritis, the *synovium*, or joint lining, may become inflamed and painful. This inflammation causes the body to produce *cytokines*, a type of protein, and *enzymes* that lead to more cartilage damage. As the cartilage wears down, the bones underneath it are exposed and can rub against each other. The ends of the bones may thicken and form growths known as *spurs*. Fragments of bone or cartilage may chip off and float around the joint cavity, causing further pain.

In osteoarthritis, there also may be changes in the joint's *synovial fluid*, which is made up mostly of a thick substance called *hyaluronan*. This fluid acts to lubricate, cushion and protect the joint – almost like a car's shock absorbers. Without enough hyaluronan, there may be more cartilage breakdown and pain.

Osteoarthritis symptoms may worsen after you overuse joints, or after periods where you use them very little. If you have OA, it's important to strike a balance between overexertion and inactivity, and get regular exercise to keep muscles strong enough to support your damaged joints. Weakened muscles, particularly those around weight-bearing joints like the knee, can cause OA or worsen existing damage in the joint.

As with most forms of arthritis, the cause or causes of OA are not completely clear. There are a number of possible causes. These include heredity (osteoarthritis may be due to a gene defect in some families), obesity (excess weight can stress joints), injury (joints are less stable after an injury) or overuse (high-level athletes often develop OA after years of repetitive strain). Because some of these causes may stem from behavior, osteoarthritis is one form of arthritis that may be preventable. For example, weight control may reduce harmful stress on your knee joints that can lead to osteoarthritis later in life.

Rheumatoid Arthritis

Rheumatoid arthritis, or RA, is another common form of arthritis. RA causes inflammation of the lining of the joints, called the *synovium*, and sometimes, in other organs of the body. Swelling, pain, stiffness and limited mobility result. Rheumatoid arthritis affects approximately 1.3 million Americans, and tends to strike women three times more often than men. The disease can begin at any age, even early childhood, but the majority of people with RA have the onset of their disease in their 20s and 30s.

Rheumatoid arthritis can be a debilitating disease. Pain and inflammation can be severe. Joints may be visibly deformed. Many people with RA experience flares (temporary periods of heightened disease symptoms) that make almost any activity, even walking across the room, painful or impossible. People with rheumatoid arthritis also may experience other symptoms such as fatigue, and an overall ill feeling that is similar to the flu.

Rheumatoid arthritis generally affects the same joints on both sides of the body. For example, both wrists may be affected, not just one wrist. RA commonly affects the joints of the hand, elbows, shoulders, neck, hips, knees, ankles and feet.

It is unknown exactly what causes RA, but we do know that unlike osteoarthritis, rheumatoid arthritis is an *autoimmune disease*, or a disease in which the body's immune system doesn't work properly. The body's normal defenses against disease turn against the body instead, attacking joints and other organs and causing irreversible damage.

Rheumatoid arthritis may be treated through a variety of drug therapies, including *corticosteriods, disease-modifying antirheumatic drugs* (DMARDs) and the powerful biologic response modifiers. In addition to drug therapy, people with rheumatoid arthritis must self-manage their disease and its many symptoms. A healthy diet, regular exercise and working cooperatively with health-care professionals are all important components in the self-management of rheumatoid arthritis. Joint protection is key for the person with RA, as many ordinary activities can cause pain and further damage to weakened joints.

Fibromyalgia

Fibromyalgia is a common, though often misunderstood, syndrome that involves muscle pain and tenderness, fatigue and sleeplessness. Fibromyalgia affects more than 5 million Americans, the majority of them female. Fibromyalgia affects children and teenagers in addition to adults.

Although fibromyalgia may cause muscle pain and aches, it does not cause inflammation or joint damage. Therefore, this condition is not really a form of arthritis but a related syndrome, a form of soft-tissue rheumatism. Fibromyalgia's cause is unknown. Diagnosis of fibromyalgia can be made only through a careful history and physical examination, not by laboratory tests such as blood work or X-rays. Fibromyalgia patients have a history of widespread pain that lasts at least three months, and pain in at least 11 of 18 *tender points*, which are specific places in the body associated with tenderness and pain.

People with fibromyalgia may experience severe fatigue, sleeping difficulties, headaches, changes in mood and sometimes, depression. Other common symptoms or related problems include alternating constipation and diarrhea, bladder irritability, abdominal pain and bloating. It is not clear what causes fibromyalgia pain or these other symptoms. But some new research suggests that people with the syndrome may have abnormal levels of various body chemicals that are involved in transmitting pain signals to the brain.

Fibromyalgia syndrome is treated through a combination of medications, including *analgesics* (pain-killing drugs) and *antidepressants*, and self-management techniques designed to help people with arthritis cope with pain, fatigue and depression.

Gout

Gout is a form of arthritis marked by sudden, intense pain in a joint, frequently the big toe. This pain is accompanied by tenderness, redness and inflammation of the joint. While gout usually affects the big toe, a condition called *podagra*, it also can affect other joints such as the knee, foot, ankle, wrist, hand and elbow. However, developing gout in one joint does not mean that a person will get it in another joint.

Gout affects about 3 million Americans, typically men in early middle age. There is an increasing number of postmenopausal women developing gout as well. Gout once was called the "disease of kings" or "rich man's disease" because it was thought that a rich diet of some foods, such as lobster and red wine, caused gout. The truth is much more complex.

The pain and swelling of gout is caused by a build-up of a chemical called *uric acid* in the blood, which deposits as crystals in the joints and other tissues. These tiny crystals can cause intense pain.

Uric acid is formed when the body breaks down waste products called *purines*. In people with gout, the body produces an excess of uric acid, which the kidneys cannot eliminate quickly enough or completely. Uric acid crystals also can form large deposits in the joints and surrounding tissues called *tophi* (pronounced TOE-fy), which can cause joint damage if not treated. Uric acid crystals also can form stones in the kidneys, leading to pain and urinary problems.

Several effective gout medications can help control the pain and inflammation of a gout flare. But in managing gout, a healthy diet also is key. Diets rich in uric acid – such foods as shellfish, organ meats, sardines, alcoholic beverages and others – can trigger a gout attack. Obesity may be linked to high uric acid levels in the blood. People with gout who are overweight should develop a weight-loss plan with their physicians, and anyone with gout should discuss their diet with a physician to make sure they are cutting back on potentially harmful foods and alcoholic beverages. People with gout probably can eat any food in moderation, but an excess of foods high in uric acid may cause a flare. Your physician may recommend a consultation with a nutritionist also.

Lupus

Lupus is an inflammatory autoimmune disease. There are several forms of lupus, the most common being systemic lupus erythematosus, or SLE. Other forms of lupus include discoid lupus, a chronic, scarring skin disease, and drug-induced lupus, in which symptoms often subside when the drug causing symptoms is stopped.

In SLE, organs of different body systems may be involved, including joints, muscles, the skin and internal organs such as the kidneys or brain. Lupus affects approximately 239,000 Americans and is more prevalent among women and in the African-American population. Lupus often affects women in their child-bearing years from the late teens to mid-40s, but it also may affect people of other ages, including children.

The exact cause of lupus is unknown. In lupus, the immune system malfunctions, mistaking the body's own cells for threatening foreign cells. Antibodies produced by the immune system attack the body's tissue by mistake. The results are arthritis, internal inflammation and organ damage.

Common symptoms of lupus include a butterfly-shaped, red rash across the bridge of the nose and the cheeks; small, scaly sores on the face, neck and/or chest; sensitivity to sun or other ultraviolet light; *ulcers* or sores inside the nose or mouth, including the tongue; pain, stiffness and swelling in the joints; *serositis*, or an inflammation of the linings of the heart, lungs or abdomen, causing pain and possibly shortness of breath; kidney problems such as *edema*, or a loss of kidney function; problems with the central nervous system; blood problems, such as *anemia*, or low red blood cell production; immune system problems, such as increased susceptibility to infections; and the presence of certain antibodies called antinuclear antibodies, which attack the body's own cells.

In addition, people with lupus may experience such symptoms as fever, fatigue, unusual sensitivity to cold in the extremities, muscle aches, swollen glands, hair loss and other signs that help doctors diagnose this complex disease. Lupus may be treated with such drugs as NSAIDs, which reduce inflammation; immunosuppressive drugs, which help block the activity of the body's immune system; and corticosteriods, such as prednisone, which also reduce inflammation.

Osteoporosis

Osteoporosis literally means when bone (*osteo*) becomes porous (*porosis*) and, therefore, brittle and more susceptible to breaks. Osteoporosis affects as many as 44 million Americans, the majority of whom are women and seniors.

People with osteoporosis may not be aware that they have the condition until a bone breaks, or until they notice reduced height or a rounding of the upper back. Diagnostic tools include physical examinations, such as laboratory tests to check blood and urine. A physician also will use X-rays and imaging studies, such as ultrasound and DEXA, to examine bone density and confirm a diagnosis of osteoporosis.

While osteoporosis tends to develop in later years, many factors that can lead to the development of osteoporosis occur decades earlier. For example, people whose diets are low in calcium-rich foods may be more susceptible to osteoporosis. In order to help prevent the development of osteoporosis, nutritionists strongly recommend a diet that includes such calcium-rich foods as milk, green vegetables, calcium-enriched orange juice or cereals, and calcium supplements. People with thin or small frames may be more likely to develop this disease. People who have an inflammatory form of arthritis, such as RA or lupus, are at increased risk, as are those treated with medications like glucocorticoids, which reduce bone strength.

Women are more likely to develop osteoporosis as they age, because their bones are 20 percent to 30 percent less dense than men's bones.

For women after menopause, lowered estrogen levels are a major factor in osteoporosis development.

Besides getting enough calcium, other self-management techniques and behavior modifications can lower the risk of osteoporosis. Avoiding smoking and excessive alcohol consumption can help prevent the reduction of bone mass. Regular exercise, including a combination of aerobic and weight-bearing exercises, can help maintain bone mass. For post-menopausal women, estrogen therapy may help keep calcium in the bones and prevent the onset of osteoporosis.

Back Pain

Back pain is a common health problem, affecting 50 percent to 80 percent of the adult population in the United States at some time in their lives. Back pain affects both men and women of all ages. Back pain is a leading cause of disability and lost work time. Estimated medical costs for treatment of back pain problems reach as much as $50 billion each year.

Back pain ranges from mild to severe. Severe back pain can greatly limit a person's activity. Most back pain is caused by an irritation of the *disc*, the cushion between the vertebrae in the spine. Discs act as shock absorbers, protecting the vertebrae from wearing out as they move. Ruptured or herniated discs are a common cause of back pain, often causing pain that spreads to the legs or feet.

Although back pain often stems from an injury or strain of the back, even a mild exertion can lead to back strain, causing pain and limited mobility. Other causes of back pain include osteoarthritis, spinal stenosis (in which the spinal cord narrows) and ankylosing spondylitis (see later in this chapter).

Most back pain is diagnosed through a medical history and physical exam. Sometimes, a doctor needs further tests to determine the cause of back pain, such as X-rays or other imaging techniques.

Treatments for back pain include rest, heat treatments such as hot showers or heating pads, and medications such as NSAIDs. In some cases, surgery is also necessary. Back pain may be aggravated by several lifestyle factors, including excess weight, stress, poor posture and lack of physical fitness. Therefore, it's important for a person who suffers from back pain to self-manage their condition through diet, regular exercise to strengthen back and stomach muscles and improve posture, and stress-reduction methods. Learning proper techniques for such common activities as lifting, carrying and sitting is also important for improving posture and reducing strain on muscles.

Ankylosing Spondylitis

Ankylosing spondylitis (AS) is a type of arthritis that primarily affects the joints of the spine and back. In ankylosing spondylitis, the joints and ligaments that normally allow the back to move become inflamed, causing pain and stiffness.

Ankylosing spondylitis is more common among men, and appears most frequently between the ages of 16 and 30. Women also develop the disease, often with milder symptoms. More than 350,000 Americans have ankylosing spondylitis. The cause of AS is unknown, but genes and heredity are believed to play a role in its development.

In ankylosing spondylitis, inflammation usually begins in the lower back and develops slowly, over weeks or even months. Eventually, inflammation associated with AS may cause vertebrae to fuse or grow together, causing the spine or neck to lose flexibility and become rigid. If the rib cage fuses, the chest cannot expand and breathing can be difficult.

Other joints involved in AS are the neck, shoulders, hips and knees. AS is a systemic disease, like rheumatoid arthritis and lupus, meaning it can affect other organs of the body as well. In addition to pain and inflammation, symptoms of AS may include fever, loss of appetite, fatigue and inflammation of the lungs, heart or eyes (a condition called *iritis*).

Physicians diagnose AS through a physical examination, a discussion of symptoms, and X-rays. A doctor may also perform a blood test to see if the patient has the gene HLA-B27, which is present in 90 percent of people with ankylosing spondylitis.

AS is treated with medications, including NSAIDs or DMARDs, such as sulfasalazine and methotrexate, which may reduce inflammation and slow or halt progression of the disease. It's also important for people with AS to maintain good posture and learn proper body position for activities like sleeping, sitting or walking. Assistive devices may help a person with AS perform common activities like grooming or dressing, particularly if joints are fused.

Bursitis and Tendinitis

Bursitis and tendinitis are common conditions that also are known as soft tissue rheumatic syndromes. These conditions are characterized by pain and inflammation in the structures and tissues around the joints. Bursitis is an irritation or inflammation of the *bursa*, a small sac located between bone and muscle, skin or tendon that allows for smooth movement between these structures. Tendinitis is an irritation or inflammation of the *tendon*, a cord that attaches muscle to bone.

In bursitis and tendinitis, pain occurs near joints, so some people may mistake this pain for that of arthritis. But arthritis is the inflammation of the joint itself, not the structures around the joint. Bursitis and tendinitis may result from overuse or injury to the joint areas, incorrect posture, stress on soft tissues due to an abnormal or poorly positioned joint or bone (such as arthritis in that joint), other diseases or conditions (such as rheumatoid arthritis or gout) or infection. A physical examination and medical history will help a doctor make a diagnosis of bursitis or tendinitis.

Soft tissue rheumatic syndromes may go away over time. Treatments for these conditions focus on reducing pain and inflammation, and include rest, heat and cold treatments, splints, medications, and physical and occupational therapy. Bursitis and tendinitis may be prevented by avoiding or modifying activities that can trigger the conditions. Poor posture, lack of flexibility and prolonged, repeated use of a joint may lead to these conditions, so regular exercise and learning proper techniques for performing common activities may help prevent bursitis and tendinitis from occurring.

Many other arthritis-related diseases and syndromes can weaken joints, reduce bone mass and increase the risk for injury, pain, fatigue and other problems. For all of these conditions, protecting joints is important. Modifying ordinary activities or using assistive devices will help you perform basic tasks more safely. In the next chapter, we'll discuss briefly why common activities can put your joints at risk, how self-management can help you stay healthy and fit, and how to find and use helpful assistive devices.

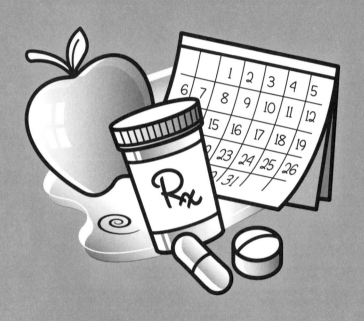

TAKING CARE OF YOURSELF:
Self-Management *and* Joint Protection

As explained in Chapter One, a successful self-manager is a person who takes control of his or her arthritis care and overall health. Why is self-management so important? Why can't you just let your doctor prescribe medication and let the pills do all the work?

Why Be a Self-Manager?

Unfortunately, arthritis symptoms can't be cured by a magic pill. Arthritis is a condition that requires your participation in ongoing care. Taking your medications as prescribed will almost certainly alleviate your pain and may slow the progression of your arthritis in some cases. But there are many other things you can and should do to ease your symptoms and prevent further joint damage.

When you have arthritis, daily activities may put your joints at risk for damage. Simple activities, such as putting groceries into your car, can be difficult or painful when you have arthritis. Lifting and carrying the groceries can put stress on your arms, wrists and back. Unlocking and opening the car door or trunk can be treacherous to hands and wrists. Lowering the heavy bags into the storage space can further strain your back, arms, shoulders and hands.

How can you go about your normal routine without putting your joints in peril each step of the way? There may be times when your activities do cause pain or minor injury, but by learning new ways to go about these tasks – one of the key components of good self-management – you may be able to protect your joints.

Joint protection is an important practice to adopt if you are going to be a successful self-manager. Joint protection involves following guidelines that help you reduce strain on your joints from ordinary activities. By following these guidelines, you reduce your chances of injury, pain, inflammation and other problems.

One of the first guidelines in joint protection is to ask for help when you need it. You may be able to ask a supermarket clerk to carry your bags to the car and put them in the trunk. You may be able to ask your neighbor to help you get the bags out of the car when you get home.

Another way to protect joints is to **use assistive devices**. You might use a fold-up, rolling cart that fits in your car as a helpful tool for carrying groceries to and from your car. To reach items on the higher shelves without asking for help, you might use a *reacher*, a long-handled grabbing tool. These assistive devices can be purchased at many stores and through special catalogs and Web sites.

When you're trying to protect your joints, it's important to **adapt your activities**. Something as simple as requesting paper grocery bags, instead of plastic bags, may be more suitable for your needs. Learning a more appropriate way to lift and carry bags of groceries may protect your arms, shoulders, back, wrists and other joints. This book contains tips of this nature to help you look at ordinary tasks in a new way, overcoming obstacles that may hurt your joints.

Your doctor, nurse, physical therapist or occupational therapist may be able to suggest new, safer ways to perform basic activities. In addition, you can learn what postures and positions cause you pain and adapt your movements to suit your particular situation. Using these approaches may help you stay independent and reduce your pain.

BASIC JOINT PROTECTION TIPS

Respect your pain. Pain is a signal from your body that something is wrong. Arthritis causes some chronic pain, but when you have sudden, excessive pain after an activity, you may be performing the activity incorrectly or may have overexerted yourself. Learn your limits and take extra care when you are experiencing pain.

Avoid improper positions. Using good posture and performing activities in the right way will help protect your joints. For example, don't slouch in a chair – keep your head, neck and back straight, your hips and knees at a 90-degree angle, your legs uncrossed and your feet flat on the floor. This will help you reduce unnecessary pain.

Avoid staying in the same position too long. Taking frequent stretch breaks will reduce joint stiffness and pain. If you work at a computer, walk around your office space every half hour, and periodically stretch your hands and fingers during typing. During car trips, take periodic breaks at tourist sites or rest areas to stretch your joints. If your arthritis is more severe, then rest breaks need to be more frequent.

- **Use your bigger joints and muscles for exerting tasks.** Knuckles and fingers can be delicate when you have arthritis. Use your palms to push yourself up from a chair or toilet seat. Carry a shopping bag by holding it in your arms, not by grasping the handle with your fingers and letting it hang.

- **Use assistive devices.** Specially-designed tools called assistive devices can help you perform basic activities. Long-handled reachers, playing-card holders, padded cooking utensils and other items can be ordered through catalogs and Web sites and purchased at many stores. You can make your own assistive devices by adapting household items to your needs. Splints and braces also may help support weak joints when you perform certain activities or when you are in pain.

- **Maintain muscle strength and joint range of motion.** Stay fit and exercise regularly to build muscles and keep joints moving well. Range of motion refers to the full spectrum through which your joint can move.

Why Fitness and Health Help Your Joints

Staying physically fit and healthy – or getting that way if necessary – is an important way to protect joints. Strong, fit muscles support joints more effectively, protect joints from undue strain and injury, and help you perform everyday tasks more efficiently and with less pain.

When you're experiencing arthritis pain, exercise may be the last thing you want to do. But if you don't exercise and move your joints, your pain will only increase. Not moving your joints makes them more stiff and painful. Inactivity makes the muscles supporting the joints even weaker, and weak muscles can't protect the joint or compensate for the joint's limited motion.

Such ordinary activities as raking leaves or washing dishes – tasks that once were just a little more difficult because of arthritis pain – may become impossible if you don't exercise. You may feel more limited by your arthritis, leading to lowered self-esteem and feelings of depression. This unfortunate cycle only leads to more pain.

EXERCISE WITH ARTHRITIS

If you have arthritis, you can and should exercise regularly in order to keep muscles and other parts of the body strong and healthy. The

Arthritis Foundation has a number of books, brochures, videos and programs designed to help the person with arthritis, as well as family members who don't have the disease, exercise safely. These exercise programs include routines for the pool or simple ways to walk for fitness.

Even simple activities, such as walking several times a week, can keep your joints, muscles, heart and lungs operating more efficiently. The Foundation publishes a helpful guidebook for developing your own walking routine, *Walk With Ease*, available by calling **800/283-7800** or ordering through the Foundation's Web site, **www.arthritis.org**. The Foundation also produces a number of exercise videos you can use at home to build strength and aerobic fitness.

In addition, the Arthritis Foundation Web site offers abundant information on exercise, diet, joint protection and other topics.

The Arthritis Foundation chapter serving your area can guide you to exercise classes in your area specifically designed for people with arthritis. Classes include water aerobics that take place in heated pools, which are more comfortable for your joints, and gymnasium exercise programs that are designed for your needs. To find the chapter near you, or to find free brochures about exercising with arthritis, call **800/568-4045** or visit **www.arthritis.org**.

WEIGHT LOSS AND YOUR JOINTS

Achieving and maintaining a healthy weight is an important part of self-managing your arthritis. Excess weight increases your risk of developing osteoarthritis, and being overweight leads to greater pain and immobility once you have the disease. For any form of arthritis, extra pounds cause additional strain on already weakened joints. Overweight people tend to be less active, leading to deconditioned muscles and more joint pain. In addition, having a healthy, balanced diet can help keep your energy level up and reduce fatigue.

Diet may be linked to the development or aggravation of certain forms of arthritis, including gout. There may be an association between a lack of vitamins and the progression of knee osteoarthritis and osteoporosis. Achieving a healthy, balanced diet is good for your joint health and overall well-being.

If you need to lose weight, do so gradually. People who lose weight rapidly on so-called "fad diets" tend to gain back their weight once the diet ends. Losing weight by eliminating certain foods or food groups from the diet, or by attempting to stick to a strict, low-calorie diet that excludes many of your favorite foods, may cause you to give up and feel discouraged. In addition, diets that promote weight loss through eliminating whole food groups may lower your intake of important nutrients.

Many people struggle with weight loss. They find it difficult to lose excess pounds, keep them off or choose a successful, tolerable diet plan. The best approach to weight loss is to consult your doctor, a nurse, a *nutritionist* or a *dietician*, health professionals who study the effects of diet, to find a plan that works for you. A health-care professional will understand the needs and challenges of a person with arthritis and help you lose weight safely and healthfully.

Incorporating regular exercise with your diet will aid your weight loss and help you keep the pounds off once you lose them. Your health-care professional can help you choose an exercise plan and can monitor your progress.

Resources for Joint-Protection Tips

When you have arthritis, your joints already may have some irreversible damage, but you can take action to prevent further damage to those joints. As we stated earlier in this chapter, health-care professionals can suggest new ways to approach common activities. This book contains hundreds of useful tips that can guide you toward more joint-friendly techniques for every type of activity.

In addition, there are many other resources available that can help you learn joint protection. The Arthritis Foundation offers helpful, free brochures on managing your activities and managing your pain, as well as an interactive Web site, **www.arthritis.org,** with useful information on managing all aspects of your arthritis. To contact the chapter nearest you, log on to the Web site or call **800/568-4045.**

Assistive Devices

Some tasks that you once took for granted may become difficult due to arthritis. Everything from holding playing cards or even getting up from the toilet seat might now be painful, difficult or impossible. It can be frustrating to need help from your family to do the things you have always done on your own.

In addition to finding new ways to go about your daily routines, you may wish to use assistive devices, or specially designed products that can make activities easier to do. Assistive devices come in many forms. Some people with arthritis may need a cane to assist them with walking and climbing stairs. Others find such appliances as jar openers, playing-card holders and zipper pulls helpful.

Many products for the home, car or office are *ergonomically* designed. This term means that the product is designed for easier, more pain-free use. For example, some computer keyboards are designed with the letters in a spread-out formation that's easier on typing hands.

Many companies produce devices specifically for people with physical limitations, and you can purchase these items in a number of ways. Ask your doctor, physical therapist or occupational therapist to refer you to sources of assistive devices. The staff at your local Arthritis Foundation chapter may be able to suggest sources for these items. At the end of this book, you'll find a list of companies that sell assistive devices, although this list is by no means complete.

Often, an assistive device is something that wasn't originally designed for that use – something you adapted to help you perform your task. You may be able to make your own assistive devices by using items you have around the house in a new way. You might wrap a towel around the handle of a bucket to make it easier to carry, for example.

This book contains many tips on how to make your own assistive devices. Making your own devices out of household objects may save money. Thinking creatively may be the best way to adapt your daily activities and household chores to your needs.

One of the most useful self-management strategies is to speak up when you need help. Your family members, friends, neighbors and co-workers may be able to help you at times when you cannot perform a task yourself. It's OK to ask for assistance when you need it, and the information on the following pages suggests ways to approach others and ways to show appreciation.

ASKING FOR HELP

It's important to remember that you cannot do everything yourself. Sometimes, in order to manage your arthritis, you must ask others to pitch in. You can delegate certain tasks that may be too difficult or painful for you.

At first, it may be awkward to ask for help. The effects of arthritis are not always visible to others, and you may be afraid that co-workers and acquaintances will think you are lazy. If you've always viewed yourself as proudly independent, this change may bother you. Try the following tips when asking others for help.

- Be specific when you ask for help. Let people know the precise task you need them to do so they can plan their schedules and not be inconvenienced. For example, if you ask your sister-in-law to drive you to the pharmacy, don't say, "Can you drive me to do some errands sometime later this week?" Let her know ahead of time where you need to go, what day, and when and where she can pick you up. Being specific shows her that you realize her time is valuable.

* Build a circle of helpers. Don't call the same friend over and over to help you with every task. Create a list of friends and family members who are willing to help you. Note what type of assistance they can give you, at what times they are usually available, and all their contact information, such as phone numbers or e-mail addresses.

* Swap help with others. One way to ask for help without feeling burdensome is to find ways you can help your friend in return. If your neighbor agrees to help you go to the supermarket every Friday afternoon, perhaps you can walk her children to the pool one afternoon a week in exchange.

The rest of this book contains just what the title promises – hundreds of tips for good living with arthritis. These tips are arranged to follow the course of a normal day. They begin as you start your day, wake up, shower, get dressed and make your breakfast. More tips follow you to work, to your daily appointments and shopping. There are tips for cooking dinner for yourself and your family, cleaning the house, paying bills, doing yard work, playing outdoor sports, unwinding in front of the TV and much more.

Tips for Good Living With Arthritis is designed to offer you helpful suggestions on getting through your day without causing unnecessary pain and strain on your joints and muscles. The hundreds of tips contained in this book are just the beginning. You may come up with more ideas on your own, adapting your own activities to your particular needs. We hope these tips will guide you and help you achieve good living with arthritis.

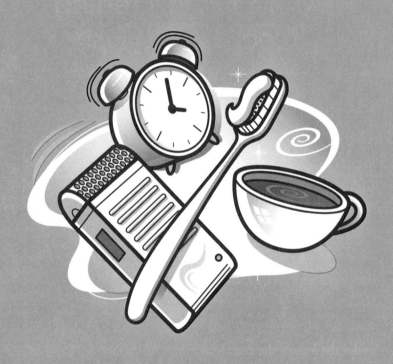

When You're Getting
Ready *for the* Day

Getting Out of Bed

⚰ If getting out of bed is difficult for you, push yourself up with your palms laid flat on the mattress surface. This leverage will give you the proper support as you stand up. Don't push on your knuckles.

⚰ As you rise, you may want to lean on a sturdy piece of furniture such as a strong headboard, nightstand or chair.

⚰ Consider elevating your bed by placing 1-inch to 2-inch blocks under the legs of the bed. Make sure the blocks are large enough – at least three times the width of the bed legs – to accommodate any sliding of the bed. Consider purchasing a higher bed.

- Keep canes or other walking aids close to your bed so you can use them when you need them.

- Place folded-up eyeglasses on your nightstand, where you can reach them without fumbling.

- If you have difficulty opening a folded pair of eyeglasses, place opened eyeglasses on top of a cloth on your nightstand so they don't slide off the table as you grab them.

- If you use a wheelchair, make sure it's the same height as your bed to ease the transition from bed to chair.

- As you get out of bed, be careful not to trip on rumpled sheets or blankets that slipped to the floor during the night. Push covers away from your feet and legs as you move to get out of bed.

- If you wear contact lenses, keep a pair of eyeglasses by the bed so you can wear them as you move from bedroom to bathroom to put in your lenses. Poor vision, especially in the morning, may lead to a misstep, trip, slip or fall.

Making the Bed

× Make your bed one half at a time.

× Use a large, lightweight bedspread, comforter or coverlet that can be slipped easily over your sheets. You don't have to tuck sheets under your mattress – just smooth them out and throw the comforter over them.

× Use a wooden pizza paddle to help you tuck in sheets and blankets.

× Attach *Velcro* to the corners of sheets to help you fasten them without having to tuck them under your mattress. Make a "hospital corner" and see where sheets need the attachments.

× As you make your bed, use a long-handled reacher to help you move pillows, blankets and sheets that are more than an arm's length away.

- To make it easier to access your pills and remember to take them each day, remove pills from their containers and put them in a seven-day pill sorter. Place the pills you take each day of the week in the appropriate section of the container. Place this lightweight container by your bed or sink so you remember to take your pills each day. Or, slip it in your purse or pocket as you leave for the day.

Toilet and Bathroom Safety

- Try a raised toilet seat if you have difficulty getting on and off the toilet. This may make it easier for you to lower yourself to the toilet seat, because you won't have to go as far.

- If you shower while sitting in a chair in the stall, consider installing a portable, hand-held shower head. These attachments allow you to move the water around your body to the places you need to wash. Select hand-held shower heads that are lightweight and comfortable to hold.

- Before purchasing any toilet or bathroom appliance modifications, make sure you measure and examine the appliance you already have. A raised toilet seat attachment for a round seat won't fit an oval or elongated style.

* Extension levers can be attached to toilet flushers to make them easier to reach and flush. You can make your own extension by attaching a wooden ruler to the flusher with heavy-duty tape. Use your elbow or forearm to push the lever down if it's too difficult to reach with your hand.

* Keep a roll of toilet paper within reach of your toilet so you don't have to get up to find one. Try placing a roll on the back of the toilet tank or on a nearby shelf.

* If you're in a wheelchair, make sure any exposed pipes in your bathroom, especially those under the sink, are properly insulated to protect your legs from burns.

Bathing and Showering

* Try other handy items for washing your body, such as long-handled brushes, shower puffs with nylon rope handles and

curved brushes that let you wash your back without stretching your arms uncomfortably.

✕ Instead of a washcloth, use a shower mitt made of terry cloth or loofah. If you sew or know someone who does, make these mitts out of an old towel.

✕ Handrails beside the bathtub and toilet and in the shower can protect you from slips and falls when you are using these facilities. Consider installing these items in your home.

✕ Use a transfer bench to slide into the bathtub more easily. You can sit down and slide yourself into the bathtub without having to step in and sit down. Use your palms to push yourself along the bench. Don't lean on your knuckles.

✕ Don't lean on a towel bar or soap dish holder for support as you are getting out of the shower or bathtub. These items are not designed to support your body weight. Install a handrail instead, or have one professionally installed.

- When showering, sit on a sturdy, waterproof chair in your shower stall. This type of chair is available at many home supply stores. You also can use a sturdy, all-weather garden chair.

- If you have difficulty turning on sink, shower or bathtub faucets, consider using a tap turner (similar to a wrench, with a long handle) or a plastic gripper that fits around the faucet handle.

- Try not to keep too many items, such as shampoos, sponges and bubble bath, stored in the bathtub or shower. Store only what you think you will use.

- Use a shower caddy, a shelf that hangs from the shower faucet, to store bath items. Caddies also place items such as shampoos, conditioners and shaving creams at a comfortable height to reach when you're in the shower.

- Do not store your razor in the shower or bathtub. Razors can easily slide off the shelf, and may cause you to step on the blade, or slip on the razor and fall.

- During a shower, use a soap on a rope, liquid soaps or body washes from pump dispensers to avoid dropping bars of soap in the shower, which can lead to dangerous slips.

- Put a rubber mat on the floor of the shower or bathtub, or stick rubberized decals on the bathtub or shower floor to keep from slipping. Buy these mats at supermarkets, pharmacies, hardware stores and discount stores.

- If it's painful for you to stand in the shower barefoot, use specially designed shower shoes. Some of these shoes slip on, or have *Velcro* ankle straps to keep them in place. These shoes also can be used at the pool or beach.

Dental Care

- Use your elbow or the heel of your hand to squeeze remaining toothpaste out of the tube. Press on the end of the tube gently to squeeze enough paste out of the opening, or use a toothpaste squeeze key or tube-squeezer device.

- If a toothbrush is difficult to grip, try wrapping the handle with the tube of a large sponge hair roller to make a fatter, more comfortable grip.

- Try using an electric toothbrush. These models vibrate the bristles back and forth over your teeth and gums, saving your hands and wrists a lot of effort.

- Stand-up, pump-style toothpaste dispensers may be easier to operate than tubes. Press down on the top of the dispenser with the heel of your hand.

- If you struggle with holding dental floss, purchase a dental floss holder at your pharmacy. These devices hold the floss in place for you while you clean between teeth.

- Electric tooth-cleaning devices, such as the *Water-Pik*, use water to clean between teeth and on the gum line. These tools may be easier to use than floss.

Grooming

* If spray anti-perspirant cans are difficult to use, try a stick or roll-on variety.

* Use lightweight hair dryers to reduce strain on hands and wrists. Try a travel-sized model for everyday use. Consider purchasing a standing hair dryer, as many salons use. You can sit in a chair under these dryers.

* To make trimming fingernails or toenails easier, soak hands and feet beforehand to soften nails. Trim nails soon after a bath or shower, or after you have been in the pool.

* If you have immune-system problems, reduce your risk of hair-follicle infections by shaving legs in a downward direction, from knee to foot, instead of upward.

* If you find an emery board hard to use, try gluing it to a large sponge and using the sponge as a holder. Just run the emery

board surface across your nails. Or, tape or glue the board to any flat surface and run your nails across the file.

* Try an electric manicure tool if you find nail files difficult to hold. Some of these tools have attachments that file, buff and clean your nails. Consider paying for a manicure and pedicure when you need nail care.

* Spring-loaded nail clippers may be easier to hold and squeeze than cuticle or nail scissors.

* Sit down to comb your hair or perform other grooming. Use a bathroom stool or keep a chair handy to wheel into the bathroom when you need it.

* If you don't have room for a seat in front of your bathroom mirror, there are mirrors that hook around your neck and allow you to groom wherever you can sit down. This type of mirror leaves your hands free to fix hair or straighten a tie.

- Use long-handled combs and brushes that allow you to groom your hair without lifting your arms. You also can attach a comb or brush to a long piece of tubing, wrapping the handle with bubble wrap to make it easy to grasp.

- To reduce joint pain and fatigue, use both hands for grooming tasks such as holding a brush, using an electric razor or brushing your teeth.

- If you find it difficult to grasp and hold grooming items like hairbrushes, select models with built-up handles. You can adapt grooming items by adding the foam tube of a hair curler or by wrapping foam or bubble wrap around the handle.

- If twisting a lipstick up and down in the tube is difficult for you, consider purchasing a thick lip pencil. You can color in your lips without having to twist a tube.

- If you prefer a traditional blade razor, find one with a large grip. Many manufacturers now make razors designed for women that have larger, easy-to-hold grips. Men can use these models, too. The razor blades are the same in both types. Only the razors' packaging and color are different.

⚔ Leave off the tops of shaving cream, deodorant or hairspray cans. Although the cans look neater with the tops on, these tops can be very difficult to push on and pull off.

⚔ If you find it difficult to hold a can of shaving cream and press the dispenser button, place the can on a flat surface. Use the heel of one hand to press the dispenser, and your other hand to hold the dispensed cream.

⚔ Consider purchasing an electric razor. Choose a lightweight model with a large grip. Some models can be used in wet environments, letting you shave while seated in a chair in your shower.

⚔ If shaving legs or underarms in the shower is a struggle, try placing a sturdy shower chair or a waterproof garden chair in the stall. Sit down while you shave.

- Shave legs while seated on a chair in your bathroom. Simply use a wet washcloth to dampen your legs, then use the same cloth to wipe off excess shaving cream. Place the chair by your sink so you can rinse the razor if necessary.

- Keep grooming routines as simple as possible. Ask your hairstylist to suggest a haircut or style that is easy to maintain.

- If your hands and fingers are affected by arthritis, don't try to trim nose or ear hairs or pluck eyebrows. Grasping small tweezers or grooming scissors can be difficult, and you may cut yourself. Ask your barber or hairstylist to perform these tasks. There also are day spas that offer these grooming services.

Getting Dressed

- Keep your closet organized so that oft-used items are easy to find. Sort your clothes by color or type. Hang sport shirts in one place, followed by pants, skirts or other items. By organizing, you won't have to dig through a batch of clothing just to find what you need.

- Install hooks on the back of a closet door to hang frequently worn hats, mufflers, belts or bags.

- Try using a canvas shoe bag that hangs on the back of a door to store shoes you wear most often. These bags allow you to access shoes without stooping, and they take up little closet space.

- Use a long-handled shoehorn to help you put on tightly fitting shoes. Make one by taping a shoehorn to the end of a yardstick.

- Use pulling attachments to make zipping and unzipping clothes easier. These pullers are large rings or tabs that hang from zippers and make them easier to grip.

- Clothes with roomier cuts in sleeves, pants legs or skirts may be easier to put on, wear and remove. Make sure you can put on and remove clothing with comfort and ease.

- Avoid clothes that require a great deal of care. Choose wash-and-wear items made of fabrics that resist wrinkling and shrinking.

- Don't overload suit or jacket pockets, which can make garments heavy and uncomfortable. Put some items into pants pockets, and consider wearing a snap-on waist pack to carry items more comfortably.

- Use dressing aids to help you put on shirts, jackets, pants and other items. To make your own, attach hooks to dowel sticks to help you slip a jacket over your shoulder or to take an item down from a closet bar without having to strain.

- Use a buttonhook to help you fasten buttons on shirts and jackets. These dressing aids consist of a metal loop attached to a grip handle. Make sure the grip is large enough to hold comfortably. Find these aids through assistive device catalogs or have a friend help you make one.

- When getting dressed for the day, choose clothing and footwear that will be comfortable and practical for your day's plans. Check the weather report before you get dressed. Dress accordingly –

and change your plans, when possible – if the weather makes it difficult to get around.

- If you have a fused neck or spine, or limited joint mobility, use long-handled shoehorns and sock grippers to help you put on your shoes and socks without bending over.

- Choose pants and skirts with elastic waistbands, which allow you to pull clothing on and off without struggling with buttons and zippers.

- Wear shoes that are sturdy and supportive of ankles and feet. Make sure they have nonskid soles, particularly for walking on linoleum, tile, waxed or wood floors.

- New leather shoes often have very slippery soles, particularly for walking on carpeted floors. Run a piece of sandpaper lightly across the sole a few times, or scuff the sole on concrete pavement, to create a less slippery surface.

- Avoid wearing clothes that are too long. Excess hem may lead to tripping and falling. Hem clothes to the correct length, or cuff pants so they don't drag on the ground.

- Use a shoe polisher that sits on the floor, rather than the small hand brushes that may be difficult to hold. Electric models polish and buff shoes without requiring you to bend or stoop. To avoid losing your balance, make sure you grasp a railing or sturdy chair when you polish shoes.

- Take care when wearing athletic shoes. The bottoms may grip carpeting, causing falls or injury. These shoes may be best for exercise only.

- Choose bras that hook in the front rather than in the back. To wear a back-hooking bra, put it on backwards, hooking it in front of your body, and then turn the hooks to the back of your body.

- Wear jackets that zip up rather than button. Attach a zipper pull if needed.

- Sit down when putting on socks, pants, underwear and hosiery. Don't try to stand on one leg to slip on these items. Sit on the edge of your bed or put a sturdy chair in your bedroom or dressing area for this purpose.

- Instead of storing socks rolled into balls, lay them flat in pairs. This reduces the need to pry apart rolled-up socks.

- Organize rows of socks in like colors, so you don't have to dig through your drawer to find the right pair.

- Use knee-high stockings under pants or long skirts instead of full-length hosiery.

- Socks made from wool and silk blends or synthetic stretch material will not slide down into shoes as easily as other kinds.

- Put shoes or clothes that are off-season – such as sandals in January or heavy sweaters in July – in the back of your closet or in a storage closet or container. Storing items when you are not using them will keep your closet more organized and make it easier to grab the items you need.

- Don't hang too many items in your closet. An overstuffed closet makes it difficult to move clothing. Try putting little-used clothing in drawers or storage boxes instead.

Making Breakfast

- Microwave ovens save time and energy in the morning. You can cook eggs in a microwave egg poacher or prepare frozen breakfasts in the microwave. The lightweight, plastic cooking pans used in microwaves are easier to hold and carry than metal cookware.

- Cook bacon or sausage in the microwave instead of in a skillet on the stove. Place the bacon strips or sausages between two paper towels to cut down on grease.

- Use a microwave that sits on the countertop at arm level, rather than a model mounted beneath your cabinets.

- Loop a scarf or bandanna through your refrigerator door handle to make it easier to open in the morning. Open the door by sticking your arm through the loop, pulling with your forearm.

- Cut bagels with a "guillotine" bagel cutter instead of trying to hold them in one hand and slice them with a knife. Drop the bagel in the slot and push down on the top of the slicer with your forearm or elbow.

- If you have trouble slicing bagels at home, ask the clerk at the bagel shop to slice your bagels for you. Freeze and store the sliced bagels in a large, resealable plastic bag.

- If boxes are hard to open, store cereal in plastic pitchers with handles. Pour the cereal through the spout or lift off the top of the pitcher and pour.

- Choose breakfast foods that don't require a lot of cooking or clean-up. Frozen waffles, pre-chopped fruit salads, cottage cheese or muffins provide a good breakfast that doesn't require slicing, frying or cleaning pots and pans. Add a glass of milk or juice to balance the nutrition of the meal.

- Buy milk in plastic containers that have twist-off tops, instead of cartons or bottles that have tops that need to be pried off. If you have difficulty twisting off a top, use a rubber jar gripper.

- If you buy milk in a carton, open it by pushing the sides of the spout back with the heels of your hands, then pull the center of the spout forward with a knife or letter opener.

- Large containers of milk, juice or other beverages may be economical, yet too heavy to carry and handle. Consider buying smaller containers, or have someone transfer the contents to smaller, lightweight, refillable containers. You also can purchase handles that fit around beverage containers to make it easier for you to carry them and pour.

- If you're preparing breakfast for the whole family, cut down on preparation and crowding in the kitchen by choosing foods that everyone likes. If possible, share cooking duties with other family members so you don't carry the whole workload.

⚹ Buy brands of English muffins that are pre-sliced.

Child Care

⚹ If you have arthritis and need to help your children dress in the morning, sit on a chair and have the child stand in front of you. This puts you both at the same height and makes dressing easier.

⚹ Choose matching outfits for your child ahead of time so that finding the right clothing will be easier in the mornings. Select clothes that will be easy for you to put on your child. Many children's clothes and shoes come with *Velcro* straps and closures.

⚹ As soon as children are old enough, teach them to do such daily tasks as putting school books in a backpack, washing or dressing. Taking on these responsibilities will feel like an accomplishment to the child and ease your morning workload.

- Bathe children in the evening rather than the morning. This way, you can bathe yourself in the morning without having to rush to see that your children are washed up, too.

- Use caution when transferring children into a car seat or the back of a car or van. Carry children in your arms, with their arms around your shoulders. Don't let children hang from your neck, or try to lift them using just your hands. If possible, push them to the car in a stroller and let them climb into the car.

- Pack children's lunches the evening before, or pack several days' worth at once. Store these meals in paper sacks in the refrigerator if the items are perishable. Advance preparation cuts down on morning rush.

- Try prepackaged kids' lunches available at your supermarket, such as crackers, cheese, luncheon meats and mini-pizzas. Consider these meals for children who are old enough to open and assemble them without help.

- Many children like drinking juice from a drink box, but these packages may be difficult for you to open. If your child is not old enough to open the drink box himself, serve your child juice in a colorful cup with a lid and a straw.

Packing for the Day

- Don't pack a lunch that is too heavy for you to carry. Use a lightweight, zippered, insulated lunch pack that can be carried on your shoulder with a strap. Pack lunch items in sealed bags or plastic containers.

- Close plastic containers by pushing down on the lid with your elbow, not by trying to seal them with your fingers and thumbs.

- Don't try to carry too much to the car at once. It's better to make more than one trip to the car, ask a family member to help you, or use a wagon or wheeled cart to carry items to the car. Store the cart in the garage, or if it's a folding model, store it in your car until you return home.

- Use a shoulder bag with a built-in wallet. These bags have slots for a driver's license, credit cards and cash, allowing you to combine your wallet items with other items you carry during the day.

- Use a briefcase with a shoulder strap, or pack your work in a backpack. If you have a laptop computer to carry, use a computer carrier with a shoulder strap.

- Look for a shoulder bag or a backpack that has a slot for a folding umbrella, so you won't have to carry it in addition to your other items.

- Use a lightweight umbrella with a push-button opener instead of a traditional model. Use both hands to grip the handle and push the button with the heels of your hands.

- If possible, don't make appointments that are very early in the morning, leaving you little time for grooming, dressing and eating breakfast. Allow enough time to get ready without being rushed. Rushing can lead to doing a task the wrong way and injuring yourself.

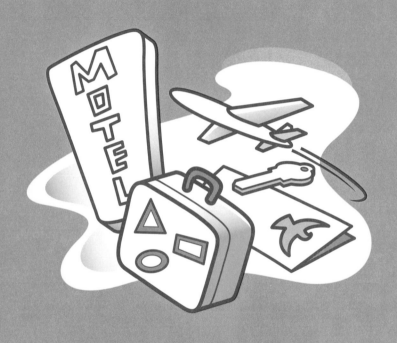

When You're On *the* Road

Driving and Parking

⚵ If you do not already have a handicapped-parking license plate or pass, speak to your doctor immediately about getting one. Handicapped-accessible parking is closer to entrances and exits, and usually is adjacent to a ramp that doesn't require you to step onto a sidewalk.

⚵ Get a handicapped-parking pass that hangs from your rear-view mirror. Take it with you if you are riding in another person's car or if you borrow a car so you will be able to park in the appropriate spaces.

- Keep your car seat at an appropriate position to support your back and neck. Insert a backrest or lumbar-support cushion if your seat does not adjust to a properly supportive position.

- If you have trouble lifting your car's door handle, try using a special lever manufactured for this purpose. This device lets you open the door using your outstretched palm, rather than your fingers.

- If you have difficulty grasping a steering wheel, consider purchasing a vinyl steering-wheel cover, which provides cushioning and makes the wheel easier to grip.

- Put your car key in a stiff sleeve that allows you to turn it with your palm or a fist instead of grasping it with your fingers. These sleeves are available through assistive-device companies, or you can make your own out of stiff cardboard.

- If you have trouble gripping a steering wheel or gear shift, use golf, baseball or weight-lifting gloves when you drive.

- Turning your car key may be difficult if the key's handle is too small. Consider having a copy made with a large, plastic handle that's easier to grip. Ask your car dealership if it can provide such a key.

- Build up the handle of a car key with thick tape or foam padding to make it easier to grip.

- To get in and out of cars more easily, use a twirling seat attachment. These seats are available through many assistive-device catalogs. To get into a car, sit down on the seat first with your legs outside the car. Pivot your body around, putting one leg then the other into the car. To get out of the car, do the reverse. Bring your legs out of the car, one at a time, first, then pivot your body and stand up.

- Choose a car by testing how easily you can access and operate it. Before you buy, get in and out of the car, adjust seats, steering wheel and mirrors, and open and close the trunk. Look for cars with automatic seat belts, which don't require you to pull seat belts across you and fasten them by hand.

* Many new cars come with key-chain controls that allow you open the trunk and unlock the doors with just a push of a button. Use the heel of your hand to push the buttons of the control, or use both thumbs.

* If you have difficulty getting in and out of your car, attach a plastic handle to the top of the doorway so you can grip the handle as you raise yourself out of or settle into the car.

* Keep a book-style road map in your car. These models are easier to use than standard maps and require less folding. Attach thick pieces of electrical tape to the ends of the pages to make it easier to flip through the book.

* It's easier to move around in cars with vinyl or leather upholstery. If you have a car with cloth seats, consider putting in a vinyl seat covering.

* If you have difficulty turning your head to look in a rear-view mirror, consider installing a wide-angle mirror. If your car has

sport mirrors mounted on both sides of the exterior, adjust these mirrors to the proper angle so that you can use them as you drive.

⚔ Keep your car free of unnecessary items to reduce the chance of tripping when you get in and out. Install a small trash bin designed for car use on the back of your seat, and empty the bin when you get home or stop by the gas station.

⚔ If your windshield is coated with ice, scraping it off may be difficult. Use a spray ice remover or set the defroster to its highest temperature. After a few minutes, the ice should melt sufficiently for you to remove it.

Walking

⚔ Wear comfortable shoes with flexible, non-sticky soles that absorb shocks. When your feet hit the ground repeatedly, you will want to have good support for your ankles and knees. Walking shoes should have arch supports, cushioned insoles and enough room in the tips for your toes.

- Try on a selection of walking shoes at the shoe store. Take the time to walk around the showroom floor a few times to see if the shoe is both supportive and comfortable. Discuss the merits of different brands and styles with the salesperson.

- When you shop for shoes, wear the same socks you use for walking, so you can find shoes with the correct fit.

- Make sure you wear socks that don't slide down into the heel of your shoe as you walk. Look for walking socks that conform properly to the shape of your foot. Ask the staff at your local shoe store or sporting-goods store to recommend walking socks.

Carrying

- Try not to carry too many items with you as you walk. Use a waist or fanny pack to carry keys, wallet, identification or other necessities. Don't pack so many items that the load becomes too heavy.

- If you're carrying a bundle to your car, hold it in your arms with your arms wrapped around it. Don't lower items like shopping bags, grocery bags, briefcases or laundry bags into your trunk using your hands. Hold bundles in your arms and bend your knees to lower them into the trunk.

* Carry purses on your shoulder, hanging across your body. Don't grab a purse by the handle and let it hang from your fingers. Use purses with shoulder straps instead of clutch or short-handled styles.

* If you are walking from your car or office to another destination, lock items that you don't need in your trunk or desk drawer so that you won't have so much to carry.

* Keep a large laundry basket in your trunk, attached to the floor with electrical tape. Put your grocery bags or other items in the basket so they don't spill or slide to the rear of the trunk when you drive, making them more difficult to retrieve.

* Keep a folding, wheeled cart in your car to transport items from the car more easily.

Cell Phones

- Having a cell phone is important for many people, whether for business, personal needs or safety. Look for a phone that is lightweight, with buttons that are large enough to dial easily.

- Cell phone clips that fit onto belts or waistbands allow you to carry a phone while you work, do household chores or run errands.

- Don't use a handheld cell phone while you drive. Driving with only one hand on the wheel puts strain on your hands, arms and shoulders. Either pull over and use the phone while parked, or put the phone in a mounted holder and use the speaker setting.

Traveling

- When making hotel reservations, ask if the hotel has a handicapped-accessible room. Many larger hotels now have such rooms, with showers, bathtubs, toilets, sinks and closets that are easier to access. A travel agent may be able to locate a hotel that can accommodate your needs.

- Always bring a lightweight carry-on bag to hold your medications, a change of underwear and socks, a toothbrush and other vital items. If you are stranded en route, because of bad weather or a missed connection, you may not have access to your checked luggage.

- When making your flight reservations, find out whether the airline can accommodate your needs. You may want to arrange assistance in boarding and exiting the plane, request that a wheelchair be waiting for you at the gate, or board and exit the plane before other passengers.

- If you prefer to sit in an aisle seat so that you can get up to stretch or move around more easily, ask for one when you are making your reservations. When you check in, remind the gate official that you reserved an aisle seat.

- During a flight, try exercising in your seat. Roll your shoulders in a circle, and flex your ankles, hands and fingers. Whenever possible, walk up and down the aisle or to the restroom.

- Avoid getting dehydrated during a flight. Bring a bottle of water with you so you do not have to wait for the flight attendant's cart. Staying hydrated during a flight may help prevent fatigue and reduce pain.

- When traveling, use a small, compartmented pill container to organize your daily medications. Keep the container in your purse, carry-on bag or suit pocket where you won't lose it and can access it easily during your trip.

- If you are traveling to a different time zone, particularly overseas, keep a log of when you need to take your medications. Take an extra watch with you that is set to your home time, so that you can take your pills at the appropriate time. If the watch has an alarm, set it for dosage times.

- Plan ahead so you won't depend on the contents of the flight attendant's cart for a snack. This strategy works for train, bus and car trips, too. Bring a piece of fresh fruit or some peanut butter crackers. Avoid salty peanuts and caffeinated drinks, which can dehydrate you or keep you revved-up, leading to fatigue.

- Consider purchasing a suitcase with rolling wheels and a pull-up handle. Suitcases that must be lifted and bags with shoulder straps can cause serious pain and strain. If you have difficulty carrying luggage, rent a rolling luggage cart, or ask the airline if someone can assist you.

- Lifting carry-on bags into overhead compartments can be difficult and dangerous for your joints. If you must put bags in the overhead compartment, let the airline attendants know that you need help or ask other passengers to help you. Consider checking heavy or bulky baggage.

- If you are taking a long car trip, plan periodic stops at rest areas. Get out of the car, stretch and have a snack. Schedule these stops and figure them into the total travel time.

- Even if you normally don't use a lumbar support pillow or backrest in your car, use one on a long car trip. Your back will feel better if it's well-supported. Take the pillow on bus, train and airline trips too.

- Make sure you can stretch your legs while in the car. If you are sitting in the passenger seat, keep it pushed back far enough to stretch out your legs. If you are sitting in the back seat, make sure there is enough room to stretch in front of you.

- If you are traveling by train or bus, take opportunities to walk up and down the aisle or passageway. Use caution when you walk, due to the movement of the bus or train. If possible, hold on to a railing while you walk.

- Many buses and passenger trains have handicapped-accessible entrances. Ask beforehand if you can get assistance with boarding or exiting.

- A train case may be a good item to have with you on a bus, train or airline trip. This case holds your essential toiletry items, and can be held on your lap or on a tray table while you sit. Often, these cases have a mirror inside the lid. Use the case instead of standing at a shaky bathroom mirror on a bus, train or airplane. Carry the case by putting it inside a tote bag with a shoulder strap.

* Travel-sized items may be convenient, but they can be hard to use. Few are adapted for people with special needs. Make room for your full-sized toiletry items or see if you can find travel-sized toiletry items in assistive-device catalogs.

* Don't wait until the last minute to pack for a trip. Plan out beforehand what you will need. Take clothing items that can be mixed and matched to cut down on the amount you pack in your suitcase. A suitcase with fewer items is easier to carry, and clothing stays fresher.

* Ship gifts or heavy items home from a trip, rather than carrying them in your suitcase. If you buy gifts or decorative items, many stores will ship them for you free or for a small charge. If you don't need an item urgently, and you can afford to ship it, this tactic may make your return trip easier.

At the Gas Station

* Don't make a trip to the gas station a painful experience. Consider using full-service stations. This service costs more, but it may be

worthwhile to let someone else fill up your tank, especially if you are having a flare. Have the attendant check your tire pressure and oil.

* Ask your mechanic if it's possible to attach a larger handle to your oil gauge so you can grasp it more easily when you check it.

* Keep a disk-shaped, rubber jar opener handy to help you twist a gas cap off the tank. There also are gas caps that do not require you to twist them on and off. These caps have a slot that allows you to put the gas dispenser in without removing the cap.

* Use both hands to grab a gas dispenser and pump the gas. Most gas dispensers have a lever that can be turned over to hold the dispenser in place while the gas pumps, so you don't have to hold it the entire time. If you have trouble with this mechanism, ask another customer or a gas station attendant to help you.

* Make sure your windshield-wiper fluid is filled at all times. It may be difficult for you to reach across your windshield to clean a spot

or remove a piece of debris. Keep a reacher or a long-handled sponge in your car to remove items trapped in windshield wipers.

× If you have to lift windshield wipers – to remove branches or trapped debris, for example – use a plastic wedge to lift the wiper slightly, then use your outstretched hand to push it up all the way.

× Keep a small, folding stool in the back of your car so you can sit while checking your tire pressure, filling your tires with air, vacuuming your car floors or pumping gas.

When You're *at* Work

Workplace Safety

⚹ Always use handrails to help you move safely and avoid injury. If your workplace does not have handrails installed, speak to your supervisor or human resources department about the possibility of adding these to your workplace.

⚹ If you work in a retail store and must stand behind a counter for hours at a time, see if your supervisor will let you sit on a tall barstool. Sitting on a stool will keep you at the customer's eye level but allow you to relieve your feet, knees and legs from the strain of standing for hours.

- If your job takes you into a warehouse setting, use caution as you reach for items on high or low shelves. If possible, use a reacher to grab inaccessible items, instead of stooping or stretching.

- Don't try to lift boxes that are too heavy. Ask someone for help with this task. Injuring yourself will only impair your ability to do your job. Take breaks during or between tasks, before you get tired. A ratio of 10 minutes of rest to 50 minutes of activity works well for many people. When your arthritis is more active, rest more frequently, for longer periods. Perhaps there are some tasks that you can do while seated, resting your limbs.

- Use coffee breaks for short walks around the office. It's important to stretch your legs and joints when your job requires hours of sitting.

- Alternate light and heavy tasks, doing the toughest jobs when you're feeling best. Don't try to reorganize your desk when you're having a flare. This task can wait for a day when you're feeling better.

Avoiding Fatigue and Pain

× Stick to the time you've allotted for work. At times, you may have to stay longer to get your job done. But if a task can wait until the next day, leave it until then. You'll get more done in the long run if you don't wear yourself out.

× Don't rush. You'll be more efficient working at a comfortable pace than at a hectic one that invites mistakes and accidents. Schedule time for the unexpected.

× Discuss with your supervisor the possibility of adjusting your work schedule. You may be able to come to work later and leave later, allowing you extra time in the morning to take a warm bath or to stretch.

× Talk to your fellow workers about swapping duties when possible. When you're having a flare, it may be too difficult for you to do certain tasks, and you may be able to trade for less strenuous duties.

- Rest your wrists and hands often. Take a few moments occasionally to rest from typing. Perform periodic stretching exercises to keep wrists, hands and fingers loose and limber.

- Alternate tasks to reduce the pressure on your wrists. If possible, type for intervals of no more than 30 minutes. During breaks from typing, file or return phone calls.

- Store your most-used items at arm level so you don't have to bend or stoop to get them. Store these items in easily accessible areas.

Office Equipment

- Lightweight plastic stacking bins with openings that are tilted downward, like a spout, make it easier to reach files, newspapers and magazines, papers and office supplies.

- Learn your photocopier's features. Instead of lifting a heavy or stubborn lid, it may be possible to place paper to be copied in an automatic feed tray. Many photocopiers also sort, stack and staple items.

- Some common office tasks, such as replacing staples in a stapler or putting fresh paper into a printer or photocopier, may be difficult for you to do. If you have trouble doing these tasks, let your supervisor know why. See if you can find easier ways to accomplish these tasks, or if you can trade tasks with other workers.

- Instead of storing copier paper in its original wrapping, store loose paper on a shelf or in an open bin. This storage will make the paper easier to access.

Using the Phone

- Don't cradle the telephone receiver between your ear and shoulder. To protect your neck and shoulders, keep your head up and hold the receiver with your hand.

- If you do hold the receiver between head and neck, attach a cradle to the receiver. The cradle lets you hold the phone on your shoulder while cocking your head only slightly.

- If gripping a phone receiver is painful, attach a handle to the receiver. Make sure that that the handle is adjusted to fit your hand size. Slip your hand through the opening and let the phone rest in your palm.

- Use a headset telephone instead of a traditional receiver. These attachments fit over your head so you can talk, but leave your hands free to type, take notes or flip through files.

- Use your phone's speaker setting when you can. This mode leaves your hands free while you converse with the other person, and it is useful for conference calls.

- Keep a pad and an easy-grip pen by your telephone so that you can write down important messages without having to scramble to locate a piece of paper.

- Talk to your office manager about the possibility of your company providing adaptive devices for your desk, such as a telephone with larger buttons. These items may make it easier for you to perform your job, increasing overall efficiency.

Writing

* Pens specially designed for people with arthritis make writing an easier task. There are models that slip over a finger, eliminating the need to grasp at all, some with molded or cushioned grips, and others that are mounted on grips at the proper angle for writing. Look for these pens and other writing tools in self-help catalogs and stores.

* If you don't have an easy-to-grip pen, add a plastic grip to your standard pen, or make your own grip with a foam curler tube or layers of electrical tape.

* Use pens that require less pressure to write, such as ballpoints, rolling points and felt tips. Avoid fountain pens, which have to be dragged across the paper.

* If you are in a class or a business meeting, using a small tape recorder is a good alternative to taking notes by hand. Make sure to keep a few extra batteries with you in case the tape recorder stalls.

- A dry-erase board is useful for writing reminders or lists. These boards come with fat pens that are easy to grip. The boards wipe clean, eliminating paper waste.

- Keep paper from sliding while you write by using a clipboard, a pad of paper or a paperweight placed at the top of the page.

Using a Computer

- When using a computer, make sure you have a comfortable chair with good low-back support and arm rests. Position your wrists so that they are in line with your forearms. Lean forward at your hips instead of bending at the waist or neck.

- Make sure the computer monitor is at the correct height. The top of the screen should be just below eye level. Readjust the height of the chair or find a chair that is the proper height.

- Lumbar support is important when sitting at the computer. Use a chair with adjustable lumbar support, or place a lumbar pillow or rolled-up towel behind the small of your back, against the chair back.

- Arrange your work area or computer so your wrists are in a natural, comfortable position. Use an adjustable chair that can be raised or lowered to the proper position. Your wrists should not be bent too sharply when you type.

- Purchase and install a keyboard tray, which places the keyboard at a more comfortable angle and level. Use a wrist rest, which extends out from your keyboard to keep your wrists elevated as you type.

- Create your own wrist rest with two strips of bubble-wrap packing material taped together. Make the bottom strip wider than the top one, and tape the excess width to the bottom of your keyboard so the wrist rest extends outward.

- If your child has arthritis, make sure his or her wrists are supported by foam or gel padding, or clip-on wrist supports. Mini-keyboards are available for children with severely limited range of motion in their hands. Also available are on-screen keyboard programs and programs that use a joystick, instead of the more difficult mouse.

- Store computer diskettes in a container that is easy to access. Some models pop the diskettes up in a fan when you open it, allowing you to select the right one without digging with your fingers. Or store diskettes in a file box with tabbed dividers.

- Jewel boxes for compact discs or CD-ROMs can be difficult to open. Store them in cardboard or plastic envelopes. To remove the disc, turn the envelope upside down and catch it with your other hand.

- If a compact disc or CD-ROM comes in a plastic-wrapped jewel box, remove the plastic with a letter opener, then pry the lid open with a letter opener or large-handled knife.

- Store contact numbers in your computer instead of a business-card holder. When you meet a new contact, type in the person's information so you can access it easily. Keep the business card in a file that you can access if your computer goes down.

- If you use a laptop computer, make sure you place it at the appropriate height. If your desk is too high, adjust your chair. If your workstation is too low, raise the laptop by placing it on a stack of telephone books.

* Make sure computer cables or other wires are not stretched across your workspace or beneath your feet when you are at your desk. Improperly stored cables can cause trips and falls.

At Your Desk

* Use turntables, lazy Susans or artists' caddies to store desk supplies, instead of putting them in a drawer.

* Use rolling carts with open shelves or bins to store papers and other office supplies. You can get what you need without opening heavy desk or file cabinet drawers, and the cart can roll with you around your workspace.

* To sit correctly, use pillows or a rolled-up towel to support your lower back. Place your hips, knees and ankles at a 90-degree angle, with a footrest, if necessary. Hold your shoulders back and tuck your chin in a comfortable position.

- If you don't have a footrest, make one out of a box of supplies, files that you don't often use, old phone directories stacked and taped together with double-sided poster tape, your kids' old encyclopedias or any rarely used items of appropriate height.

- To sit properly at your desk, your shoulders should be relaxed with your arms at your side, elbows at a 90-degree angle or lower, and your wrists straight. Use an adjustable chair if you need to position yourself for different work surfaces, such as a standard desk or counter.

- If it is difficult to sit down at or arise from the front of your desk, sit in a higher chair.

- Use a book stand to avoid neck strain when you look down to read. Book stands can be placed on a desk, table or bed tray.

- If you're typing from a written page, clip it to a raised clipboard that attaches to the side of your computer. This device, available at office-supply stores, lets you see the page without having to look down.

- If you use plastic file holders or staggered file bins to store important files on your desk, you rarely will need to struggle with heavy file drawers.

- Use a wedge-shaped calculator, rather than one that sits flat on the desk. Use trays that hold calculators in a raised position, making them easier to operate.

- Use electric staplers and pencil sharpeners to make daily clerical tasks easier on the hands.

- Keep paper clips in a magnetic holder. Shake the holder to bring paper clips to the magnetized opening. Don't keep paper clips in a box or in the tray of your desk drawer.

- Use preprinted rubber stamps for commonly used addresses. These stamps will save your hands from excess addressing and writing.

- Use large-handled scissors, instead of traditional scissors.

- Use a wheel-shaped business card holder to store important phone numbers and information. Don't overstuff the holder; keep it loose enough to flip through and easily find important information.

Mailing

- Use self-sticking stamps instead of the kind that must be torn off and moistened. If you have difficulty removing the stamps from their backing, use a letter opener.

- Office postage machines, which print postage on letters or labels, save time and energy. Postage also can be downloaded from the Internet and printed directly onto envelopes. Log on to www.usps.gov for more information.

- To moisten stamps and envelopes more easily, use a gel moistener or a slightly damp sponge, which can be stored in a plastic holder. This strategy is particularly helpful if you have Sjögren's syndrome or take medications that may cause dry mouth.

- Stack envelopes in your desk drawer with the flaps open and hooked over the next envelope. This method makes individual envelopes easier to grasp.

School

- Request a free copy of the Arthritis Foundation brochure "When Your Student Has Arthritis." Give a copy to principals and teachers at the beginning of each new school year. Set up an appointment to discuss your child's needs. Explain how and why a child with arthritis or a related condition may do things differently from the other students in the class.

- Children with arthritis should not sit in a cross-legged position. Although this is popular in many preschools, teach the child to sit with his or her knees extended.

- Find large-handled, easy-grip pens, pencils and markers for your child. These writing utensils also are good for older students and college students.

- Before the school year begins, ask the principal if special locker arrangements can be made for your child. If the school has stacked lockers, see if you can reserve one that is between waist- and shoulder-height. Ask if your child can have a locker on each floor of the school to limit carrying. Perhaps your child can share lockers with other students on each floor.

- Ask your school if it is possible to supply your child with two sets of books, one for on-campus study and the other set for home.

- Use backpacks, not bags that are carried by hand, to carry books. Backpack straps put the weight on larger joints like the shoulders, rather than straining weaker joints like the wrists and fingers. You can also use a book bag with wheels and a long, extending handle.

- Pack your child's lunch in a paper sack or a zippered, insulated pack that can be carried on the shoulder. If school meals are preferred, arrange for someone to carry the tray for your child.

- Small children with arthritis may need more time than other children to use the bathroom facilities. Ask the teacher if your child can have more time to use the bathroom, or can use it before or after the other children.

- If you are a college student with arthritis, discuss your needs with your professors. Also, contact your admissions office or student affairs department to find out if there are any special services you may be able to access. These services may include special parking stickers or housing priority.

- College students should schedule classes to limit the amount of walking or rushing between courses. Sometimes, special scheduling isn't possible and consecutive courses are located far apart. Explain your situation to professors so that you will not be penalized if you are late.

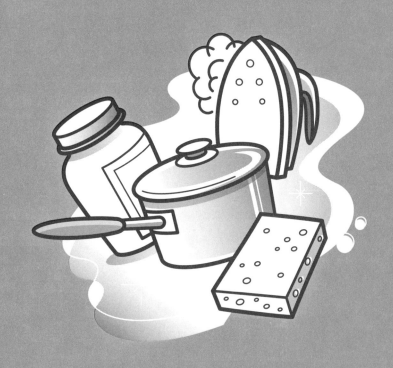

When You're Around *the* House

Moving Around

⚐ Don't leave bags, boxes, toys, laundry baskets or other items in hallways, walkways or stairways. Keep areas free of obstacles to reduce the chance of tripping or falling.

⚐ Keep electrical cords out of walkways or high-traffic areas.

⚐ Replace or remove carpeting that is frayed or loose. Carpeting on stairways that is loose can lead to trips, falls and injuries.

⚐ Consider installing handrails and grab bars in shower stalls and bathtubs and around toilets. Handrails will make using these areas easier and safer. Make sure rails are installed properly to avoid accidents and injuries.

- If the phone rings and you are not near an extension, don't run to answer it. Rushing may cause you to fall and injure yourself. Use an answering machine, voice mail or caller identification service to let you know who calls.

Carrying

- Don't grasp items too tightly. Protect your finger joints by grasping such items as tool boxes, shopping bags, baskets or handheld tools only as tightly as necessary to use them. Use built-up grips made from rubber or plastic foam on pens, eating utensils and tools.

- Always hold a tool or utensil parallel to your knuckles. Don't hold the item so that your hand is forced to twist toward the little finger.

- Carry shopping bags in your arms, not by the handles, so that you shift the weight to your larger joints and protect your more delicate hands, fingers and wrists.

- When carrying a bundle like a bag of groceries, hold it in your arms, close to your body.

- Use a utility apron with large front pockets to carry such items as cleaning supplies or tools around your house. Use the apron when you go grocery shopping to carry your wallet, keys and grocery list.

Pushing and Pulling

- To close a heavy or stubborn drawer, push it with your backside. Don't try to force a drawer shut with your hands or fingers.

- Push in dining room or kitchen chairs by using your hips or backside, rather than your hands or fingers.

- If you have to move such objects as boxes or chairs across the floor, slide them rather than picking them up and carrying them.

- Use reachers to access hard-to-reach items. These extension tools allow you to grasp, twist or pull items without having to overstretch your arms.

- Don't stand on a chair or in an opened drawer to reach a high shelf. Use reachers to grab items from high places, or stand on a sturdy stepstool.

Holiday Shopping

- Instead of filling out cards for holiday or birthday presents, order gift enclosure cards with your name printed on them. Tape these cards to the top of the gift or slip them inside the wrapped package.

- Order preprinted holiday cards with your name inside the card and your return address on the envelopes.

- Use printed address labels instead of writing your return address on holiday cards. Children can help with peeling and attaching the labels onto the envelopes.

- Office-supply stores can create a rubber stamp with your name and address on it. You can use different colors of ink to create unique return addresses on your envelopes. This stamp also can be used after the holidays.

- If you find it difficult to peel off the paper on a bow's sticky strip, attach the bow with a small piece of double-sided tape, a sticky-side-out loop of tape, or a dollop of rubber cement, which dries clear.

- Instead of wrapping boxes, use gift bags. Roll the gift in tissue paper and slide it in the bag, leaving the excess tissue poking up at the top for a festive look.

- For preparing and serving holiday meals, make a division-of-labor list for your family. Assign tasks beforehand so that everyone knows his or her duties. Let your family know that you need their help in creating a special meal for everyone.

- Make your family's holiday meal a potluck. Assign each person a dish to bring. To cut down on cleanup, tell each person to bring food in its own serving dish, which can then be taken home to wash.

- Create an assembly line in the kitchen for food preparation and clean-up. When washing dishes, one person can wash, one can rinse, one can dry and stack, and one can put away dishes.

Cleaning

* If you have a two-sided sink, fill one side with warm, soapy water. Put dirty utensils into the water to soak immediately after using them. This method makes the utensils easier to clean later. If it's inconvenient to use your sink for this purpose, fill a plastic bowl with warm, soapy water for soaking utensils.

* Put a small rubber shower mat in your sink to keep pots and pans from moving while you scrub them.

* If you have a deep sink that forces you to bend to retrieve items on the bottom, consider installing a sink rack.

* Some dishwashing brushes can be mounted on the wall by your sink or on the side of the sink. These brushes attach with suction cups and may allow you to wash cups, bottles and other dishes without holding a scrubbing brush.

* Sit while you wash dishes. Place a high chair or stool near the sink so you won't have to stoop.

- Keep fingers extended when you scrub, either with a scouring pad, a washcloth or a sponge.

- Use a rack to let dishes air-dry instead of drying them with a towel. This method saves energy and saves your hands from having to maneuver a towel.

- Place small utensils in a mesh, waterproof bag in your dishwasher to keep them from falling out of the racks and into the bottom of the machine. Baby-supply stores and grocery stores stock plastic containers designed to hold small items in the dishwasher.

- Collect laundry or paper waste by placing it in a wheeled cart. If your cart doesn't have a long handle, attach a rope or an old bathrobe belt to the basket so you can pull it around.

- Make your own wheeled cart. If your kids don't use the skateboard anymore, glue an old canvas laundry bag or a plastic laundry basket onto the board. Attach a rope or an old bathrobe belt to the front wheel axle. Pull the rolling cart from room to room.

- Vacuum by walking with your vacuum cleaner, instead of pushing and pulling it back and forth while you stand still. This method reduces stress on your arms and wrists, and can be a good aerobic exercise.

- If an upright vacuum cleaner is difficult to maneuver, consider using a canister model instead. Many canister models are lightweight and easier to carry from place to place. Use the type of vacuum cleaner that suits your needs and physical limitations.

- An all-surface carpet sweeper is a lightweight option for cleaning dirty floors and carpets. Keep the sweeper in a corner or in an accessible hall closet.

- Place rubber-bottomed doormats in front of outside doorways to reduce dirt tracked onto floors and carpets. Cutting down on dirt cuts down on vacuuming.

- Keep your fingers extended when holding a sponge for cleaning the car or washing dishes.

- Use a dustpan with a long handle, which will allow you to sweep up dust without bending. Attach the sturdy cardboard tubing from a used roll of gift wrap to a short dustpan to make a long handle. Bend the end of the tube, slip it onto the handle and tape securely with masking tape.

- To make a handy dust mop that will dust high or low places, attach your dust rag to an empty gift-wrap tube. Staple a rag to the end of the tube to reduce bending and reaching when you dust.

- Place your trash can on top of an old wooden crate or sturdy box. This method makes it easier for you to pull out the bag without having to stoop.

- Use garbage cans with wheels to make trash clean-up easier. Tie bags of garbage while they are still in the can. Then roll the can outside or down to the curb for pick-up. If you don't have a rolling garbage can, place bags in a rolling cart or wagon to take outside.

Talking on the Phone

- Look for a telephone model that has large buttons, which are easier to read and operate.

- Take the time to test models in the store before you purchase one. Make sure you are comfortable picking up, holding and replacing the receiver, and that the buttons are easy to dial.

- If you have room, place a tall stool or chair near a wall phone so you can sit comfortably while you talk.

- If possible, buy a portable phone. You can bring the receiver with you as you move around so you don't have to rush to another room just to answer the phone.

- Many phones can be programmed for speed dialing. You can store many of the numbers you dial most frequently. Some phones automatically store the telephone numbers of incoming calls, allowing one-touch call-back. Familiarize yourself with the special functions your phone offers.

* Put a magnetic, dry-erase message board and marker on the refrigerator near your kitchen phone. Write messages on the board. These boards can be wiped clean after use, eliminating paper waste.

* If you talk on a wall-mounted phone, install an extra-long extension cord. The longer cord allows you to talk on this phone while sitting on a nearby chair or leaning against a counter.

Household Tasks or Crafts

* When addressing envelopes or paying bills, work at a desk or table that provides a firm, flat surface and is at a comfortable height for your arms and hands. Don't write while sitting on your bed.

* When doing needlework or handiwork, take frequent breaks to stretch your hands and fingers, and to change the position of your neck and back. If you find that your hands become stiff or painful during your handiwork, try using a heat treatment before you start.

- If your favorite craft has become too difficult, see if there is another, similar craft that is easier on your joints. If you always liked to sew by hand, a sewing machine may be a good alternative. If you enjoyed needlepoint but can't handle the small needle anymore, you could try crochet or macramé, which use larger tools and wider yarns. Ask the clerk at your local craft store to make suggestions.

- Enlarge handles on tools, utensils, knitting needles, pencils or pens to make them easier to grip and handle. Wrap tape, bubble wrap or foam packing material around the handle so your grip won't be so tight. Purchase items with easy-to-grip handles, available at many stores and in catalogs.

- Sit when you work on your favorite craft or at a household task. If sitting is not possible, take short, frequent breaks.

- Whenever possible, transport items on a cart rather than carrying them. If you are painting a window trim in your guest room, don't try to carry paint, rollers and drop cloths. Put these items in a wheeled cart and roll them from room to room.

Entering or Exiting Rooms

* Make your home easy to enter and exit. Install a railing along entrance stairs for support and balance. If a step up to a door is too high for you to manage comfortably, create a half-step by securing a piece of wood on the bottom of the existing step.

* If your ability to walk is very limited, or you are in a wheelchair, consider having someone install a ramp at the entrance of your home. The ramp should have a handrail, a slip-proof surface and a smooth landing area. Before you install a ramp, check with your physical therapist to determine if the ramp meets the necessary standards.

* In your home, make door knobs easier to open by installing door-knob turners. These turners fit over the knob and have a handle that extends. Push on the handle with your hand or arm.

* You also can replace door knobs with models that are easier for you to open. Search your local hardware or home-improvement stores for different models, and have a professional or a friend install them.

Other Household Safety

- If pulling curtains open using the cord and pulley is difficult for you, install wands at the openings of curtains so that they can be pushed easily along the curtain rod.

- Make curtains out of lightweight materials, such as batiste, silk, sheer nylon or cotton. Heavy, woven fabrics may be more difficult for you to open and close.

- Install electric controls for shades, blinds and curtains. These controls make opening window treatments much easier on your hands and fingers.

- If your blinds have a rod that you twist to open and shut the slats, attach a thick, foam hair curler to the end of the rod to make it easier to grasp.

- Sliding doors, such as those leading to a patio or garden, may be difficult to open and shut. Ask a friend to rub the tracks of the door with liquid soap or petroleum jelly to keep them sliding smoothly.

- When having your house painted, make sure the painters keep window hinges, tracks and seams free of paint. Ask painters to leave windows open while the paint dries so that they will be easier to open later.

- To dust blinds, use a long-handled duster that reaches the higher or lower blinds without making you stoop. Open blinds partially to clean the entire surface of the slats, as well as in between.

Floor Safety

- Avoid throw rugs. You can trip over rugs, and rugs make it more difficult to move furniture. Firm, flat carpeting is preferable.

- In bathrooms, make sure bath mats have a nonslip backing, or purchase such a backing at your home decor store. If your footing is very unsteady or your mobility is very limited, consider not using bath mats.

- Tack down the edges of carpeting. A loose carpet edge, particularly near a step, can be a hazard.

- Use non-skid wax on kitchen or bathroom floors. A waxed floor can be dangerously slippery.

- When it's cold, never walk around your house in just your socks or stockings. Socks may make it easier to slip and fall. Use a supportive house shoe or go barefoot.

- Avoid running electrical cords across areas where you or others may walk. Exposed cords increase the risk of trips and falls in the house.

- Use caution when plugging in an outdoor electrical appliance, such as a leaf blower, or when using a garden hose far from the house. Let your family know that you are using the appliance, and that the hose or cord is stretched across the lawn or driveway.

- If a lamp or electrical appliance has excess cord lying on the floor, use a cord shortening reel to keep the cord neatly stored and reduce your chance of tripping and falling.

- Night lights can illuminate floors when house lights are turned off, making trips to the bathroom and other nighttime walking safer.

- If you need to transport something tall, such as a houseplant, roll it in a wheeled cart or scooter instead of trying to carry it in your arms. If you can't see around the item you're carrying, you could trip or fall over something in your path.

- If you're installing electrical outlets, don't place them too low on the wall so that you have to stoop or bend to reach them. Place outlets or telephone jacks at a comfortable height that also accommodates your electrical appliances.

- If you have trouble handling standard lamp switches, buy lamps or use converters that allow you to turn the light on and off by touching the lamp's surface. Use remote-controlled lights also.

- A simpler way to make lamp switches easier to use is to add a large, specially made knob over the existing switch. This knob makes the switch easier to grip and turn.

× If you wish to plug lamps or other items into an outlet that is hard to reach, try a multi-plug unit. These are long bars with a row of outlets that can accommodate a number of plugs. These outlets can be placed in more accessible spots. Also, pushing down on a plug may be easier for you than pressing one into a socket from the side.

× Use timers to turn lights on and off at times that are convenient for your schedule.

Stairway Safety

× Install light switches at the top and bottom of stairways, so that you do not have to climb or descend unlit stairwells.

× Cover stairs with a surface that resists slipping. If you can, install a carpet runner up the middle of a stairway. If you cannot install a runner, ask your local home improvement store to suggest an easily attached, nonskid surface that can be placed over stairs.

× Install sturdy handrails along stairs, even in places where there are just two or three steps, and use the handrails at all times.

- Always turn on the lights before you proceed up or down a stairway.

- If you cannot install light switches at both ends of a stairwell, see if there are electrical outlets at some point along the stairwell. Plug in a night light to illuminate stairs in the evening hours.

In the Kitchen

- Use waxed paper instead of plastic wrap to cover items for heating in the microwave. Waxed paper is easier to tear and handle, and it works well in microwave ovens. Waxed paper also may be used to wrap leftover luncheon meat for refrigerator storage.

- Try new plastic wrap designs that are easier to use, including disposable, plastic dish covers with elastic. These look like shower caps and fit over dishes easily.

- A slow cooker may help you prepare a meal without rushing and feeling fatigued by the experience. Buy meat already cut into chunks or have your butcher cut it for you. Put the meat, pre-chopped vegetables and water into the slow cooker. Prepare the meal early in the day when you have more energy.

- If you need to fill a large pot with water, don't fill it in the sink. Using both hands, place the pot on the stove. Then, fill a glass, small pitcher, watering can or kettle and pour water into the pot until you have the amount needed.

- When cooking small items, use a countertop toaster oven or convection oven so that you won't have to bend or stoop to put food in the oven.

- Use heat-proof gloves or mitts instead of square pads when removing hot pans from the oven. These mitts are easier to grip with, and they protect your forearms from accidental burns.

- Search kitchen catalogs or shops for items that may be easier for you to use in cooking. Look for lightweight, aluminum pans with two handles, which are easier to hold. Some lightweight pans come with broiling racks that can be used instead of the heavy, bulky broiling pan that comes with most ovens.

⋈ When washing dishes, using a mitt made of sponge material may be more comfortable than trying to hold a sponge or scouring pad. These mitts are available at hardware stores in the automotive accessories departments.

⋈ To save time and energy, cook eggs in a microwave egg poacher, or prepare frozen breakfasts that can be cooked in the microwave. The lightweight, plastic cooking pans used in microwave ovens are easy to hold and carry.

⋈ Use a microwave that sits on the countertop at arm level, rather than a model mounted beneath your cabinets, which can cause you to stretch your arms unnecessarily.

⋈ Use a microwave with a turntable feature so you don't have to turn items halfway through cooking.

- Take care not to let items cook too long in the microwave. Foods can explode and splatter if heated too much, leading to a difficult cleanup. Cover food with a paper towel or wax paper to keep the food from splattering.

- When possible, use both hands to lift pots, saucepans, bowls, pitchers or other containers. This method reduces stress on your hands and wrists. Use caution when trying to lift a hot saucepan. Remove the food from the pan using a spatula, spoon or tongs and leave the pan on the stove until it has cooled.

- To stabilize a saucepan or skillet while you stir cooking food, rest the pan's handle against a filled tea kettle on the next burner. Look for panhandle holders that attach to the stovetop with suction cups.

- Use tongs instead of a fork to turn food, such as chicken breasts, during cooking or grilling.

- Griddles with low sides may be easier to use than skillets for cooking chicken breasts, chops or fried eggs. The low sides make it easier to turn food with a spatula, or to slide it off the griddle and onto a platter.

× Use pots and pans with nonstick finishes to cut down on clean-up. Spraying the surface with cooking spray reduces sticking even more.

× When lifting or holding large bowls, pots or pans, hold your fingers straight instead of trying to grip the container to decrease stress to your hands and reduce pain.

× A convection oven that sits on your countertop may be a good alternative to using a regular oven or an oven that is mounted underneath a cabinet. These ovens bake, broil and roast, but you can slide pans in and out of them without having to bend or stoop.

× Use an electric knife for carving large roasts. Look for one with a grip that allows you to hold the handle with two hands, as electric knives tend to vibrate when they slice.

- Buy cheese already grated or shredded. These cheeses come in resealable plastic bags, and will save your hands from strenuous grating. If you have a hard time resealing these bags, close them with bag clips.

- Make opening a jar easier by stabilizing it. Place the jar on a rubber mat, then twist the top open with a rubber jar gripper. Twist the lid open by placing one hand on the side of the jar, and the heel of your hand on top. Turn the lid toward the thumb side of your hand.

- Open a jar by placing it in a shallow drawer. Close the drawer enough to squeeze the jar between drawer and countertop, then use both hands to twist the lid open. Use this method for bottles as well.

- Mount a jar opener at chest height on the kitchen wall. Let the grip of the opener hold the lid securely while you use both hand to twist the jar open. These openers also can be mounted underneath shelves and cabinets. Make sure you are able to lift your arms and hands up to open the jar.

* When making muffins, line cups with paper liners to avoid having to clean baked-on batter.

* Get the children or grandchildren in your family involved in food preparation. Children can measure sugar or spices, mix batter or wash vegetables. Cooperation will save you extra work and allow the kids to do something helpful and fun.

* Many kitchen appliances and cooking utensils come with easy-to-grip handles. Be a proactive consumer. Look for these items at your local cookware store, or ask the manager if the store can order these items for you. There also are a number of catalog and Web site companies that sell easy-to-use cooking items.

* Use pre-chopped, bagged vegetables and salad mixes to save energy when preparing meals. Bags of frozen mixed vegetables can be defrosted and used in casseroles, stir-fries, salads and omelets. Bags of frozen vegetables can double as a handy ice pack for stiff, painful joints.

- When making stir-fry, chicken salad or casseroles, use chopped, pre-cooked chicken breast, sold in the refrigerated section of many supermarkets, to save the effort of slicing chicken. Canned, cooked chicken also may be used for casseroles, chicken salad or soups.

- Store, reheat and serve leftovers in the same microwave-safe dish so you don't have to transfer food from one dish to another, and so you don't have to wash several dishes. A dinner bowl covered with plastic wrap probably takes up as much space in your refrigerator as a rubber-topped storage tub, and it keeps foods fresh.

- Keep cooking utensils within easy reach. Put the items you use most often in drawers or cabinets that don't require you to reach or stoop to open them.

- Try hanging utensils like wooden spoons or tongs from hooks underneath the kitchen cabinets. This technique keeps you from having to stoop to retrieve utensils, and from having to dig through a cluttered drawer to find them.

- Use both hands to lift or pour from any container. If using a plastic pitcher, wrap both hands around the body of the container and use the handle for support as you carry the pitcher.

- Use a butter knife or other utensil to loosen any can tops that have a ring or pull tab, or to pop open a can of soda. Don't try to pry the top open with your fingers. Place the can on a rubber mat or damp cloth to keep it from sliding.

- Don't clutter drawers or cabinets with items you never use. Give away or discard unnecessary gadgets so you don't have to dig around for what you really need.

- Keep a stable, sturdy stool in your kitchen for reaching items on top shelves. If you feel uncomfortable stepping on the stool, ask someone else to do it or to "spot" you while you step up. Try to find a stool with a handrail for easier use.

- When mixing cake batter in a stainless steel or aluminum bowl, place a rubber jar gripper underneath the bowl to help stabilize it while you blend the batter with an electric mixer. You also can put the bowl in a dry, clean sink to keep it steady, and rest your arms on the sides of the sink while you mix. Keep the electrical cord out of the sink at all times.

- Beat eggs with a lightweight, large-handled whisk rather than a spoon or fork. Using a whisk offers less resistance and will be easier on your muscles.

- When reaching for items on high shelves, use a long-handled pair of tongs as an extended gripper. Also, consider trying grippers and reachers that are available at department stores or through assistive device catalogs.

- If a jar is too difficult to twist open, use a jar key opener to release the pressure. These devices have a point on one end for opening cans of liquid and a bent metal lip on the other end. Simply wedge the pointed end underneath the lip of the jar lid, and pull up. The lid's pressure should release – you'll hear a pop – making the jar easy to open.

- If you find a jar key difficult to hold, wrap electrical tape around it to thicken the grip. You may find more easy-to-hold utensils in assistive device catalogs.

- Cut open bags of chips with a large-handled pair of kitchen scissors. Transfer the chips to a plastic bag with a sliding seal, a little plastic clip that slides back and forth easily to seal the bag. You may also use a large clip to close the bag.

- Use kitchen scissors to cut open slices of individually wrapped cheese, then pull off the plastic wrap. Large-grip scissors also can be used to cut off pats of stick butter or margarine, and chop the tops off celery stalks.

- To skim the fat off soup without constantly spooning, drop a few ice cubes in the soup and then fish them out with a ladle. The fat will cling to the ice.

- Another way to skim fat off soups is to lay lettuce leaves on the top of the soup and then pull them off with tongs. The fat will cling to the lettuce. There are also utensils, available in most kitchen specialty stores, that attract fat from soups and stews.

⚹ Learn to make "one-pot" meals to save the time and effort of cleaning a number of dishes. Stews, pasta dishes or chicken cooked with vegetables in a foil, disposable pan or oven-baking bag can make easy meals with limited cleanup.

⚹ Don't transfer a cooked dish from the pot to a serving dish. Put the pot on a heatproof trivet right on the dinner table, or put servings on the plates in the kitchen and then serve them to your guests.

⚹ If you're having family or friends over for dinner, make the meal a potluck affair. Assign each relative or guest a dish to bring so you won't have to cook the whole meal.

⚹ Use a large plastic pitcher or a bowl with a spout at one end for mixing cake batters. This method makes it easier to pour batter into the pan. Hold the pitcher or bowl with both hands when you pour.

- To keep a pan from sliding when you're pouring batter into it, place the pan on top of a slightly damp washcloth, rubber mat or kitchen towel.

- Consider using premixed, rolled cookie dough instead of making cookies from scratch. The dough can be sliced off with a knife or clipped off with large kitchen scissors. Some brands are pre-scored, which allows you to break them apart, then bake. There are new brands of cookie dough that are already formed into balls. Simply place these balls on a cookie sheet and bake.

- Large-handled pliers or nutcrackers can help loosen tightly sealed bottles. To make handles easier to grip, wrap electrical tape around them, or use the foam cylinders of old hair rollers.

- Use a long-handled meat fork to turn meats in the oven or under a low-lying broiler so you won't have to reach or stoop so far. Hold the fork with both hands if you can. Build up the fork's handle with electrical tape if you find it difficult to grasp.

- When setting the table, don't try to stack too many dishes and carry them to the table all at once. If the stack is too heavy, you may strain your fingers and wrists.

- Carry dinner plates to the table using both hands.

- Use a long match or long-handled electric lighter to light gas stoves or pilot lights. These lighters will keep you from having to bend down to light the stove.

- Slide heatproof sleeves over the long handles of pans or steaming baskets to make them easier to grasp. These sleeves also protect you from burns.

Eating

- Use utensils designed for people with arthritis. Utensils come in various, easy-to-hold styles: extended, angled, large-grip handles, swiveled and with hand straps. These utensils may make it easier for you to eat your food, with less pain and discomfort.

- If you have difficulty getting food off the plate, try plates with a curved rim. You can push the food up against the rim and scoop it up with a spoon or fork. Look for curved plates in many assistive device catalogs and in the children's department of many discount and department stores.

- To keep your plate from sliding around the table as you eat, place a damp washcloth or a rubber jar-opening disk underneath the plate.

- Use the proper utensils to cut and eat your food. Use a steak knife to cut meat instead of struggling with a dull blade. Use a large soup spoon for soups and chowders instead of a smaller spoon.

- Try a knife with a perpendicular handle that is laid flat so the handle looks like a T. Cut your food by pressing on the handle with your hand, and rocking the knife blade back and forth.

- Use a plastic mug instead of a glass for drinking. Slip your hand inside the handle and wrap it around the mug. The handle rests on the outside of your hand for extra support.

- If your hands tremble or you are concerned about dropping a mug, try a travel mug with a cover. Drink through the small hole in the mug's lid or insert a straw.

- Use a pizza cutter to cut sandwiches, chicken breasts, hamburgers, lasagna and other items. Roll the cutter back and forth across the food to slice it into bites or portions. Hold the cutter with both hands.

- Don't prepare foods that will be a struggle to cut and eat. Try hamburger patties instead of roasts or chops, and lasagna instead of spaghetti, which may be hard to twirl on your fork. Have family members pitch in with food preparation. If you're having shrimp, for example, ask someone in your family to peel the shrimp before serving so you don't have to struggle with shells when everyone else is eating.

- If you have trouble holding a heavy drinking glass, try using long, bendable straws that enable you to drink from a glass without picking it up.

- If you have limited neck motion and find that the bridge of your nose gets in the way when you drink from a cup, cut V-shaped notches in your plastic cups. Use large-handled utility scissors for the job.

Child Care

- Organize a nursery or child's room to reduce unnecessary movements. For example, keep bathing supplies near the area where you bathe the child, and keep fresh clothes near the diaper-changing area.

- Store items like wipes, diapers and towels in plastic stacking bins or drawers that are waist-high so you can access necessary items without stooping. In lower bins or drawers, store items that you use less frequently, such as clothes that the baby hasn't grown into yet.

- Try out any nursery furniture or baby equipment before you buy. Make sure you can lower, raise and lock the crib wall easily and without pain. Some crib models may be better for your joints than others. Make sure you can lift items like strollers and car seats without strain.

- Carry diaper bags slung over a shoulder, instead of carrying them with your hand by the straps, or use a lightweight backpack to carry diapers and changing items. Don't pack the bag with more items than you need.

- If your friends and relatives are giving you a shower, register for items that you have tested for joint-protection effectiveness. Ask the shower hosts to circulate a list of these items to the guests.

- Make sure you have time to rest. When your child is taking a nap, sit down and rest tired muscles and aching joints. Ask someone to watch the baby for a few hours while you nap or rest.

- Swap child-care tasks with another parent. For example, offer to babysit later in exchange for help when you are tired or experiencing a flare. You will feel as if you are providing a service in exchange for one.

- Use baby carriers that fit on your back or hang across your stomach like a sling. These models will be easier for you to lift and carry than hand-held varieties. Some baby carriers have *Velcro* attachments that allow for easy adjustment and removal.

⚞ People with fibromyalgia may have problems with sling-style baby carriers, particularly if they have tender-point pain in their shoulder. A hand-held model or folding stroller may be preferable for these people.

⚞ Choose a lightweight, folding stroller that is easy to transport in the car and to maneuver through your daily activities.

⚞ Use a long-handled reacher or grabbing tool to pick up discarded toys from the floor. Don't leave toys on the floor. Stray toys can cause dangerous trips and falls.

⚞ Place the highchair over a sheet or plastic mat to simplify clean-up.

⚞ Attach cloth shoe bags or small, plastic vegetable bins to the wall around the baby's changing table to store diapers, wipes, plastic pants and other items at a comfortable, reachable height.

- Instead of carrying the baby from room to room, place the baby in an infant seat secured to a rolling cart. A cart with shelves underneath will allow you to store items like bottles, wipes and clothing.

- When bathing a baby, choose a portable plastic tub with a drain in the bottom so you don't have to tip the tub over to drain out the water.

- When your child is old enough to bathe in the regular bathtub, sit on a low, sturdy chair or stool beside the bathtub to assist with bathing. Don't sit on the toilet or on the edge of the bathtub.

- Look for a playpen with an adjustable or raised floor to help you pick up the child without stooping or bending uncomfortably.

- Dress your infant or toddler in clothing that is easier for you to handle. Look for clothes with elastic waistbands, *Velcro* fasteners, V-neck shirts and zippers with larger pulls.

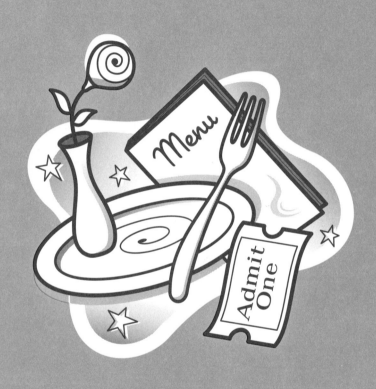

When You're
Out *and* About

Running Errands

× Avoid activities that tax you beyond endurance. For some people,
overactivity might mean the New York Marathon. For others, it's
going to the miniature golf course after you've spent a long day
of sightseeing, just because your companions think it will be fun.

× Carry a rubber, jar-opening gripper in your purse or coat pocket
and use it for grasping doorknobs.

× If you have difficulty getting on and off escalators, ask clerks,
security personnel and information desk attendants where the
elevators are located. Most malls, offices and department stores

that feature escalators also have elevators, but they may not be noticeable.

* When entering or exiting buildings or department stores, look for an automatic door or handicapped-accessible door. These doors allow you to push a large button to open the entrance, so you won't have to struggle to open a regular or revolving door.

* Consider your time and energy when you shop or run errands. Is driving an extra 15 minutes to a discount store really worth saving 50 cents on light bulbs? Your time and energy are at least as valuable as gasoline. Keep shopping short and simple.

* Carry items in a waist pack to eliminate stress on your lower back and improve posture. A home-improvement store or hardware store may stock an apron with deep pockets, which can be used to carry small purchases, wallets, keys or other items.

* When lifting or carrying a shopping purchase, use your palms instead of your fingers, and your arms rather than your hands.

* When climbing stairs in public places, step up with your stronger leg and step down using your weaker leg.

* Take advantage of free gift-wrap services when buying presents at department stores, or ask the sales clerk to wrap the item in tissue and place it in a decorative box. Top the package with a stick-on bow and you have a festive present for your loved ones.

* If holiday shopping at the mall is too stressful or difficult, consider buying gifts online or from mail-order catalogs. Ship the gift directly to the recipient. Make sure you order well in advance so your gifts will arrive in plenty of time.

* Many mail-order companies will wrap the gifts for you, so take advantage of this service if it is free or in your budget.

* If you prefer to shop for gifts in person, look for stores away from the malls, which may be less crowded. Hardware stores, supermarkets, bookstores and discount stores in strip shopping centers have holiday gifts too.

⋈ Choose one type of gift to get everyone on your list, an item that can be purchased at one store instead of 10. Books, sporting goods, clothing, videos and food items are gifts that everyone likes, and they can be individualized.

⋈ When taking children to see Santa Claus at the mall, bring a lightweight, portable folding seat with you so you can rest your legs and feet while waiting in line. Perhaps the kids can carry the seat if you don't have the energy. Some folding seats have straps that let you carry them slung over your shoulder. See Santa before you shop so you and your kids won't have packages with you in the waiting line.

⋈ Let your family and friends know ahead of time about arthritis-related gifts that you like and need. These items may include assistive devices like reachers or playing-card holders; soothing treatments like paraffin wax baths or gift certificates for massages or pool exercise classes; or offers of help to do yardwork, shopping, cleaning or other chores. These gifts may bring you more joy than another sweater or CD.

Grocery Shopping

* Use a folding, rolling cart to transport groceries to and from your home or car. Take it to the mall to help you carry your purchases.

* Ask for paper bags instead of plastic at the supermarket. These large bags can be carried more easily in your arms than plastic bags with handles.

* Even if you have just a few items to purchase, use a cart. Don't try to carry more than one item in your arms. Inquire if your store has motorized scooters for the convenience of disabled shoppers.

* Avoid using hand-held baskets, which can get very heavy with even a few items and cause pain to your hands and arms.

* Investigate using one of the new online or phone-order grocery services. Many companies now provide a wide variety of grocery and pharmacy items that can be delivered to your home. Before trying a grocery delivery service, ask your friends if they have used the service and been satisfied.

- If you wish to stay loyal to your local supermarket, ask the manager if the store has a delivery service or would consider starting one.

- Turn a trip to the supermarket into an opportunity to exercise. Push the shopping cart once around the perimeter of the store without stopping. This trick not only offers you a short walk, it gives you a chance to see what the store has on sale before you start filling the cart.

- Make sure the grocery bagger puts similar items in the same bag – refrigerated foods, fresh vegetables and fruits, sodas – so your unpacking is an easier task.

- If you think you will need assistance getting the groceries in your car, ask for help. Supermarkets will want to keep a good customer happy and safe.

- Let your store manager know that you like certain brands that have easy-to-open packaging. If the manager knows a customer will buy a certain brand, he or she is more likely to make sure the item is in stock.

- See if some of your favorite foods come in easy-to-open packaging. For example, if you find it difficult to open jars of olives, choose canned olives instead. These containers may be opened with an electric can opener, saving your hands from strain.

At the Pharmacy

- When shopping for over-the-counter medications, search for containers that are easy to open. Look for ribbed or enlarged caps that are easier to grip and turn. Some brands may advertise an "easy-open" cap. Ask your pharmacist if you can test these brands to make sure they will work for you.

- When shopping for topical analgesic creams, look for brands with flip-style caps instead of screw tops.

- Many states require that your doctor request easy-to-open containers for your prescriptions. So ask your doctor to note on your prescription that you would like your pills placed in such containers. If your pharmacy keeps customer profile information, ask the pharmacist to note your preference for easy-to-open containers.

- Avoid pill containers that require you to use your fingers to remove or replace the cap. Choose brands with tops that you can open using your whole hand or by pressing and turning with the heel of your hand.

- Look for brands of over-the-counter pills and topical creams that carry the Arthritis Foundation's "Ease-Of-Use Commendation Seal." These brands' containers have been independently tested to assure that they are easy to use for people with arthritis.

At the Barber Shop or Hair Salon

- Let your hairstylist know that you have arthritis, and that certain body movements or positions may be painful. You may need help moving and holding your head in certain positions for washing, cutting, drying or styling your hair.

- If you find it difficult to style your hair with rollers, ask your hairstylist if a permanent may achieve the same look. New types of permanents don't have the "poodle" curl look of the old varieties, and require only washing and air drying.

- At the salon, ask your hairstylist to use a towel like a sling to support your neck during your shampoo. This technique will protect your neck as you lean back over the sink and when you raise your head afterward. Some hairstylists are able to support your neck with their hands while shampooing your hair.

- Bring an inflatable pillow to the salon and place it over the edge of the shampoo sink to protect your neck. Ask your hairstylist to store this pillow at the salon for you.

- If you feel stiff during a haircut, ask your barber to stop snipping for a moment so you can shift or stretch your limbs.

Eating Out

- It's important to sit in a supportive, comfortable chair when you are dining. Ask that the host seat you at a table rather than a booth.

- Avoid restaurants that have uncomfortable or rickety chairs. Let restaurant managers know this seating is a problem and ask if chairs could be changed.

- If you are spending a long evening with family or friends at a restaurant, sitting for a long period of time may make your joints stiff. Between courses, get up and walk to the restroom or to the bar area. This tip also may keep you from nibbling too much from the contents of the bread basket.

- Bring a foam cylinder or hair curler to restaurants and keep it in your pocket or purse. Slide the tube onto forks or spoons to make the grip easier to hold. Don't forget to remove it before the waiter clears the dishes.

- If you have difficulty grasping silverware, purchase utensils with large or easy-to-grip handles. Many companies sell cutlery specifically designed for people with arthritis. Don't hesitate to bring these utensils with you to a restaurant. Put them in a resealable plastic bag and take them home to wash.

- Follow suit with glassware. Look for cups and glasses that are designed for people with arthritis, or styles that you find easier to grasp and hold. Bring these cups to your favorite restaurant.

- If you find it easier to grasp a mug with your hand inside the handle, ask the waiter or waitress to serve your beverages in one – even if you're drinking wine.

- Don't struggle with chopsticks in an Asian restaurant. Even the most authentic restaurants should have a fork available. Ask for one. To be safe, bring your own fork in a plastic bag.

- Take a little extra time to order your food. Choose items that are not only healthy, but also easier to cut and eat.

- Ask your server to bring you a large-handled steak knife to cut any type of food, not just steak. The fat handle of a steak knife may be easier to grip.

- If you have pain or limited range of motion in your hands, some foods may be difficult to cut, pick up or eat. Some examples include spaghetti, which is challenging to twirl; fajitas, which are difficult to wrap and hold; and steak and roast beef, which are hard to cut. Choose other items or find alternative ways to eat your favorite dishes.

- In a pizza restaurant, don't struggle to cut and serve your pie. Ask the server to cut the slices all the way through so you can grab them easily, or ask that the slices be cut and put on your plate.

- Cut spaghetti into smaller segments first, making it easy to spear with your fork or lift with a spoon.

- Ask your server or one of your companions if they can wrap your fajitas or moo shu rolls for you, or eat the contents with a fork and use the wrappers to sop up the sauce.

- Ask your server or one of your companions to cut your roast beef or steak for you.

- If you have the dry mouth associated with Sjögren's syndrome, running out of water during your meal could be uncomfortable. Make sure your server knows you need plenty of water to sip, or ask for an extra glass.

At the Theater

- ☒ Your joints may become stiff during a long movie. Get to the theater early, so you can choose an aisle seat or a handicapped-accessible seat that allows you to stretch your legs periodically.

- ☒ If you become uncomfortably stiff or feel pain, get up for a moment and walk to the lobby. Missing a minute of the film is preferable to being distracted by pain throughout the entire movie.

- ☒ Plan your day so you can take a hot shower or bath before leaving for the theater. A heat treatment beforehand will help your joints and muscles stay loose for the two or three hours you're sitting in your seat.

- ☒ If you bring a topical analgesic to the movie theater to rub on sore hands, arms, ankles or feet, choose an unscented variety. In close quarters, others may be distracted from the film by the odor of your cream.

- If your back becomes sore sitting in movie seats, bring a back pillow or rolled-up towel to the theater for lumbar support.

- If you have Sjögren's syndrome, bring sugar-free candies to suck on during a movie. Also, ask the concession stand for a courtesy cup of water to sip during the film.

- If you have a disorder that affects circulation, such as Raynaud's phenomenon, theaters and other large, open spaces may be cold and drafty. Bring a pair of light gloves or a muffler to wrap around your hands.

Shopping for Clothing

- If you wear splints or braces from time to time, make sure your clothing will fit comfortably over these devices.

- Always try on clothing before you purchase it, so you can determine how difficult it will be to put on and remove.

- Consider purchasing shirts with *Velcro* fasteners, which are easy to fasten and pull apart.

- Adapt your own clothing with *Velcro* tape or tabs. Use the *Velcro* to replace buttons on men's shirts, the fly of a pair of pants or hooks on front-closing bras.

- Try shirts with snaps instead of buttons for easier fastening.

- When trying on a shirt in a store, test how easily you can button and unbutton it. If you struggle now, you won't find the buttons easier to operate later on. Don't buy it.

- Avoid clothing that fastens in the back or on the side. These items may be too difficult to put on and take off.

- To save time choosing outfits and doing laundry, try to find clothing that is versatile and goes with many other items. Neutral shades, like black, gray or beige, can mix with many items in your closet.

- If a salesperson offers to help you, accept the offer. While you continue to look for more clothes, ask the salesperson to put the items you have already chosen in a dressing room. This way you don't have to carry a load of clothes around the store while you shop.

- If an item doesn't fit, ask the salesperson to bring you the item in a different size while you wait in the dressing room.

- Look for pants, dresses and skirts that are lined. Lined clothes are easier to slip on and off, and for women, lined skirts eliminate the need for a slip.

- Many clothing stores offer complimentary tailoring services. Let your tailor know you have arthritis and find out if clothing can be adapted by replacing zippers or buttons with *Velcro* fasteners.

Shopping for Shoes

- Check the *shank* of a shoe – the portion of the sole where the foot's arch is located. The shank should be rigid, providing appropriate support.

- Choose shoes with a firm, supportive *counter* – the area of the inside of the shoe curving around the back of the foot and heel, along the Achilles' tendon.

- Look for styles with a *toe box* that has room for your toes to fit comfortably, in both width and height.

- Shop for shoes with tops that are soft enough to mold around the foot. Shoe tops should not be made of a hard, unyielding material.

- Try not to select shoes that have seams around the toes and the ball of the foot. These seams can irritate your foot and cause pain.

- If you wear orthotic devices or insoles, make sure you use them when you are trying on shoes.

- If you struggle with shoe laces, try shoes with a *Velcro* closure, or choose loafers and other slip-on shoes. Try elastic shoelaces, which allow you to pull shoes on and off without untying the laces.

- Choose boots that have zippers up the leg, rather than slip-on models. These styles are easier to put on and take off. Attach a pull to the zipper to make it easier to operate.

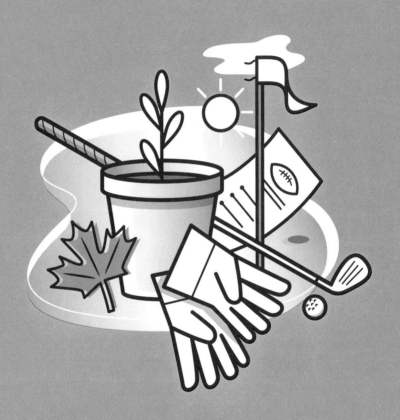

When You're Outdoors

Yard Work

* Although yard work is an enjoyable activity that provides good exercise, take care not to overexert yourself. Do what is within your limits, and ask friends and family to help.

* Use a hand truck or dolly to move heavy bags of soil, mulch or fertilizer. You can transport heavy items without having to lift them onto a cart or wagon.

* Cut open bags of soil or fertilizer with large-handled utility scissors. Don't try to rip open the plastic bags with your fingers.

- If you find it difficult to push an electric mower, consider using a riding model. If you do use a riding mower, choose one with an adjustable seat with full back support.

- If mowing the yard is too difficult for you, ask around your neighborhood to find out if someone can help you with this chore. A high school student might mow your lawn for a few extra dollars. You may want to price the services of a landscaper.

- To move around the yard while weeding or raking, use a wheeled chair or "scoot seat" designed for garden use. Use these chairs for washing and waxing the car or painting low window trims.

- If you must shovel snow, use a specially designed snow shovel with a bent handle. This device will put less stress on your back. Consider using a lightweight, electric snow blower to move snow away from walkways or driveways.

- Don't sit on the ground when you pull weeds or plant bulbs. Sit on a low step-stool or a turned-over metal basin instead. Make sure the seat is low enough that you can bend over easily to do your gardening.

× When you rise from your garden seat, place both palms flat on the seat and push your body up.

× Use your child's old wagon to carry gardening tools, bulbs or plants around the garden while you work. If you don't have one in the attic, these wagons can be purchased at toy and hardware stores.

× Use a wheeled cart or basket to carry bulbs and gardening tools around your yard. You can push the cart with your feet if you find it difficult to stoop down to move it. Tie a rope or old bathrobe belt to the basket and pull it around the yard.

× Share gardening chores with your family members or neighbors. Divide duties so you don't have to perform the more difficult tasks. Perhaps your neighbor's child or a grandchild can dig the holes, while you follow along and put the bulbs in the holes.

- Leave muddy boots or grass-covered shoes used for yard work outside the door. You'll keep mud and clippings away from your carpeting, reducing cleanup. Keep a fresh set of shoes by the door to slip on when you come back in the house.

- Don't try to cut grass on creek banks in your yard. These areas are slippery, muddy and difficult to traverse. Ask a friend or neighbor to help you mow this area, as well as hillsides and slopes.

- Search your local garden store or home-improvement center for special raised or tiered containers for growing flowers, vegetables, herbs and other plants.

- Seed tape, which can be laid in the ground or in long planters, may be easier than planting seeds by hand.

- Buy gardening tools with adaptive handles that are easy to grasp, or build up handles yourself by wrapping them with electrical tape, bubble wrap or foam padding.

- When carrying a large plant, hold it in your arms, close to your body. This technique places the weight distribution on your larger joints, such as your shoulders.

- If you like flower gardening, but can't sit on the ground or stoop to low flower beds, try planting flowers in window-box containers or clay pots that sit on tables outside your house. Consider building a greenhouse with raised shelves and tables to hold pots of flowers and plants.

Walking

- Use care when walking on a beach. Some beaches are made of soft sand that is difficult, if not impossible, for toes to grip. If the beach is made of hard-packed sand, walk on the portion that seems flattest and hardest.

- Do not walk too close to the ocean's edge, where the sand is softer and uneven. See if there is a boardwalk that will let you walk on a flat, hard surface while gazing at the ocean.

- When walking longer distances, such as in the park, to your neighbor's house, or to the store, stop for breaks. If there are benches along the way, sit down for a moment, lean up against a tree or building.

- When walking, wear loose, comfortable clothes that "breathe," such as cotton T-shirts, shorts and sweatpants, fleece pullovers or exercise clothes made from such specially-designed fabrics such as Supplex™ and polypropylene.

- Wear bright, reflective clothing when you walk. Sporting-goods stores carry reflectors that can be attached to vests or windbreakers. These attachments will reflect car headlights so you can be seen in low-visibility conditions. If possible, avoid walking during dusk or evening hours, when visibility is low.

- Don't push yourself to walk farther or faster than you feel comfortable, or up steep hills. If you find yourself becoming out of breath or dizzy, stop walking and sit down by the side of the trail until you feel better. End your walk and slowly return home or to your car.

* Dress in layers so you can pull off items, adjusting to your body's changing temperature as you walk.

* Choose your walking route with care. Scout locations before trying to walk there. Make sure the walking surface is flat, firm and level. Steep grades, uneven ground, stairs or broken pavement could lead to hip, knee or foot pain or injuries.

* Paved sidewalks, fitness trails or malls (preferably at less-popular shopping times) are good locations for safe walking. Drive around your neighborhood to find where other people walk. Your neighbors may know safe, accessible walking routes in your area.

* Ask friends or neighbors if they would like to start a walking club. Find people who walk at the same pace as you do, or close to it. Pick a convenient time for everyone. Walking with others will encourage you to keep up your routine, adds a social element to your outing, and is safer. If you fall or become injured, someone will be there to help.

- If you walk alone, consider carrying a cellular phone with you. If you fall or injure yourself, you may need to call someone for help. Use a cellular phone that clips on your belt so you won't have to carry it in your hands.

- If you walk for exercise at your local shopping center or mall, don't stop to window-shop or purchase items. You can, however, reward yourself for developing good exercise habits. For example, if you walk briskly around the mall three times without stopping, four times a week, purchase a small gift for yourself at your favorite store.

- End your week of walking by treating yourself to a healthy snack. Try a fruit smoothie or a nonfat yogurt. Don't indulge in greasy items like french fries as a reward for exercising.

- When on vacation, make time in your day for exercise. You will have more energy for sightseeing, and you'll keep your muscles and joints from getting stiff while sitting on tour buses or visiting museums.

* When you travel, pack a set of comfortable exercise clothes and shoes. Many hotels have fitness centers with treadmills or stationary bikes. Bring a bathing suit for laps in the pool before or after your day of sightseeing, or for a soak in a whirlpool bath to soothe aching muscles.

Outdoor Chores

* Use a garden hose that fits on a reel and retracts when you are done using it. The retractable reel will save you from struggling with a heavy hose, trying to wind it up and put it away.

* Use caution after watering lawns or washing your car, as the wet grass or driveway may be slippery and dangerous.

* Having a pet may help you become more active and get outdoors. If you have a dog, take it for daily walks so you both will get some fresh air and exercise.

* Ask your family members to let you know when they are using a hose. You should be told if a hose is stretched across the walk-

way, lawn or driveway. In addition, wet surfaces can be slippery and dangerous.

- Use a sturdy leash with a loop handle that is easy to grip. Avoid thin leashes and leads that are hard on your grip. Select a dog collar that is well-fitted and won't slip off when you walk your pet on a leash.

- Some breeds of dog may be too difficult for you to walk and control. Choose your pets accordingly. If your dog is overly rambunctious or hard to control, consider leaving the walking duties to someone else, such as a friend or a professional dog-walker.

- If you have a very strong or energetic dog, try putting the dog on a long lead attached to a sturdy post in your yard so it can get the proper exercise.

- If you have to clean up after your dog, use a long-handled "pooper-scooper" instead of the short varieties. These models don't require you to bend to ground level.

Sports

* Tennis rackets can be modified for easier use. Choose a light-weight racket with a larger head. There are many models made of extremely light, but durable materials. When having your racket strung, request that it be strung a bit looser to soften the impact when you hit the ball.

* Don't try to hit a one-handed backhand. Use two hands to hit your backhand. You may wish to hit your forehand shots with two hands also.

* If you find a tennis racket difficult to hold, consider building up the grip with padding, or having an extra grip added to the existing one. Use a soft rubber grip on the handle of your racket that will be easy to grasp.

* Singles tennis may be too strenuous. Consider playing doubles instead, which requires less running. If you don't have a partner, ask around at your local tennis club or in your neighborhood for someone who might need a partner.

* Swimming is an excellent exercise, indoors or outdoors, for people with arthritis. Make sure you are swimming in a heated pool with easy access in and out of the water.

* If you have your own swimming pool, install a pool ramp so getting in and out of the water will be less stressful.

* You may wish to use pool slippers for exercising in the pool or for walking around the wet pool area. These shoes are made of rubber or nylon and have strong grip soles to keep you from slipping.

* If you like bicycling, consider using a bike with a high backrest on the seat to give your back extra support as you ride.

* Bicycles with fatter wheels, such as mountain bikes, or even three-wheeled models, may offer you more balance and stability.

* Always wear a helmet when you ride a bicycle. Even a slight bump can cause a fall off a bicycle, and it's important that you wear protective gear.

- Fishing and boating can be enjoyable activities that get you outdoors. When boating or fishing, use a swivel seat similar to one that is used in your car. Adding this device will make it easier for you to turn from side to side. Sporting-goods companies manufacture such seats for boat use.

- Use the bathroom before you go boating if your boat is not equipped with a toilet. You don't want to have to go back to shore, then climb out and back into the boat, interrupting your day of fun.

- If you have a boat with a toilet facility, consider installing handrails for added stability and safety. When the boat is on the water, you may have unstable footing.

- If your boat has a manual anchor, consider installing an electric one. Manual models may be too heavy to lift and lower.

- Use a fishing vest or camping jacket to hold small items when you are fishing. These vests and jackets have numerous pockets, which usually are fastened with *Velcro*.

- Carry tackle boxes in your arms, close to your body. Don't hold a heavy tackle box by the handle and let it hang from your fingers.

- Add a supportive backrest or cushion to boat or canoe seats. Sitting on a backless seat when boating may cause strain to your muscles and joints.

- Use a fishing-rod holder to free your hands from having to hold the reel while you're waiting for a bite. There also are belts that can rest or hold your fishing reel, reducing stress on your arms.

- If you like boating but can no longer handle a sailboat, consider a cruiser or a houseboat. These boats have many comforts, such as bathrooms, and can be as easy to drive as a car. Choose a boat that is accessible and easy to operate.

- If you carry your golf bag, there are styles that can be slung across your back like a backpack. You also can carry the bag over your shoulders, bearing the weight across your body. Don't try to lift and carry the bag with your hands.

- When golfing, use a golf cart. You can get out of the cart and stretch, or walk part of the way while one of your companions drives.

- Use lightweight golf clubs instead of heavy, steel models. There are many new golf club designs with titanium shafts that are much lighter than older models.

- Find golf clubs with built-up, easy-to-grip handles, or adapt yours by adding a grip or padding to the end of the club.

- If your spine has limited mobility, or if you have had joint-replacement surgery, consult a physical therapist to discuss ways to modify your golf swing and other aspects of your golf game.

Grilling and Barbecuing

- Use both hands to carry a platter of hot dogs, hamburgers, chicken breasts or steaks out to the grill. Hold the sides of the platter or its handles with your outstretched palms. Don't clutch the sides of the platter with your fingers.

- When taking a platter of hot food back to the kitchen, use caution not to burn yourself. Use long, heatproof mitts when you hold the platter.

- Place your platter of meat on a folding table near your grill. Transfer the cooked food to the platter. Have guests line up with their plates and serve food from the grill-side table.

- If carrying a platter of food to and from the grill is too difficult, use a wheeled cart or child's wagon to roll the platter back and forth.

- If you are in charge of the grill, choose foods that you can easily flip and remove from the grill. A large Porterhouse steak may be too heavy for you to turn, and could lead to injury, burns and frustration. Try hamburgers, hot dogs, chicken breasts or lamb chops instead.

On the Patio

- Make sure your patio, back yard or deck is in good repair, with no loose boards, stones, cracked pavement or divots. These obstacles can cause dangerous trips, slips or falls, particularly for someone with limited mobility in their knees and hips.

* If you have a raised deck on the rear of your house, consider installing a ramp instead of stairs to lead down to the back yard. Deck stairs can be rickety and difficult to use. A solid ramp with sturdy handrails might allow you to use your deck and yard more easily.

* If you cannot adapt your deck with a ramp, clear a path from a ground-level door to the back yard of your house, so you can exit the house safely and gain access to the back yard. Clear away any bushes, tree limbs or roots, and fill any divots to reduce the chance of tripping and falling.

Exercise Outdoors

* A level, well-mowed back yard can be a great place for light exercise. Try kicking a ball back and forth with the children in your family, or toss a rubber ball to your dog and let him fetch it and bring it back to you.

- Croquet might be another entertaining exercise. Build up the croquet mallet handles with padding to make them easier to grip.

- Hiking can be an enjoyable and leisurely form of exercise. Investigate any hiking trails before you embark on your hike. Avoid trails with any uneven, slippery footing, steep inclines or any trails that require you to climb using your hands. Pick an easy, beginner's trail that is well-marked. Hike with friends – never alone – and bring a cellular phone and identification card with you.

- Don't overstuff your backpack if you are going on a hike. Take only what you need. Use a backpack that has a pouch to hold a water bottle so you won't have to carry it.

- Consider using a walking stick when you hike on a trail. A stick will provide extra balance and stability, and can be useful for pushing branches out of the way.

- Always wear strong, supportive shoes or hiking boots when you hike, but don't wear boots that are heavier than you will need.

Discuss the equipment you will need with your sporting-goods salesperson. Wearing an overly heavy hiking boot for a leisurely trail walk will cause strain on your legs. You may be able to hike in a good pair of walking shoes.

Outdoor Photography

* If you enjoy photography outdoors, consider using a camera with a waist harness so you can balance the camera without putting too much strain on your hands and arms.

* A lightweight, folding tripod may be useful for outdoor photography. You can rest the camera on the tripod and place it on garden walls, rocks or other surfaces. Using a tripod frees your hands to work the camera, and eliminates the need to hold and balance a heavy camera.

* Some cameras can be heavy and difficult to maneuver. You may be able to achieve the same photographic results with a smaller, more lightweight camera. Many new models have auto-focus, flash adjustment and other features that don't require you to twist

lenses and push a variety of buttons. Consider using these "point-and-click" models.

* Select a camera with drop-in film loading, not a model that requires you to pull the film strip out of the roll and feed it into the camera.

* Use a lightweight, mesh, nylon photographer's vest for outdoor photography. These vests have numerous pockets for you to carry film, lenses and other items.

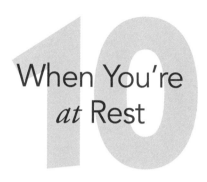

When You're
at Rest

Watching TV

⚹ While you're watching TV, get off the couch and walk around about once every 30 minutes – perhaps in between your favorite shows or during commercial breaks – to keep joints from stiffening. Don't just walk to the refrigerator and back.

⚹ Instead of just sitting in a chair or on the couch to watch TV, try folding laundry or ironing in front of the TV set so you can get a little exercise while you watch a program.

⚹ Don't watch TV while lying on the couch on your side. This position will cause neck discomfort and back pain.

* When sitting in a chair to watch TV, maintain the proper posture. Keep your feet resting flat on the floor when you are sitting all the way back in the chair. Thighs should rest comfortably on the chair's seat.

* If pushing the buttons of the remote control that came with your TV set is difficult, consider purchasing a universal remote control with larger buttons. Self-help catalogs and electronics stores may have an appropriate alternative model.

Sitting

* Staying in one position for a long time adds to stiffness and pain. Do a quick check of your jaw, neck, shoulders, arms, wrists, fingers, hips, legs, ankles and toes. Stretch and relax areas that are tired or tight.

* To achieve good sitting posture, make sure you have an appropriate chair. The back of the chair should provide firm support to keep your body from slouching. Armrests can help support your body as you rise out of the chair.

- If you use a recliner, choose one with a high back that extends to the top of your head and provides neck support. The chair's armrests should be at a comfortable height that doesn't cause shoulder hunching or slouching. Also, the recliner should allow you to adjust your position easily. Don't use a recliner that is so low that it's difficult to get out of the chair.

- Use pillows to support your neck and back as you sit in front of the TV. You can buy pillows made for this purpose, or use any small pillows that fit comfortably behind your neck without pushing the head forward, or fit in the small of your back.

- Wear comfortable clothing when you relax. When you come home from work, remove your work clothes or any clothing that is constraining or tight. Warm-up suits, sweatshirts, sweaters or elastic-waist pants are good clothes for relaxation time.

Games and Relaxation

- Although you may enjoy games like card-playing as a form of relaxation, you may struggle to hold playing cards and other items. Search assistive device catalogs for playing-card holders that keep cards in place without revealing them to your opponents. These catalogs also contain games and sporting equipment adapted to the needs of people with arthritis.

* If you have difficulty holding and tossing a pair of dice, toss the dice in a cup or mug and pour them out.

* If you find it difficult to handle playing cards or game pieces, play games with your friends or family in a team format. Divide into twos and let your partner handle cards, dice, play money or game pieces while you help with strategy.

* Keep an easy-to-grip pen or pencil handy for group games that involve drawing or writing on a large pad, or let a partner handle the writing and drawing tasks.

Bedroom

* Keep your bedroom floor free of objects that you may trip over if you get up during the night. If you remove pillows or blankets

before you go to bed, place them out of the way, on a shelf or a chair.

× Your bedroom should be a place for rest and relaxation. Don't sit on the bed to do your paperwork, writing or household chores. Save the bedroom for sleeping, sex and resting. Beds should not be used as desks, as they don't provide proper back support or an appropriately positioned writing surface.

× Keep a flashlight near your bed. Check the batteries periodically to make sure the flashlight is in working order. Having a flashlight handy can help you find your way to the bathroom during the night, without flipping on all the lights and disturbing others. If there is a power outage, having your flashlight within reach is key to your safety.

× Make sure your safety items are prepared for emergencies. Change the batteries in your flashlights and smoke detectors when you change your clocks twice a year for the daylight savings time adjustments.

- If you sit up in bed, stretch your legs out straight and use a sturdy bed tray to hold a book, a TV remote control or other small items.

- Make sure your mattress is firm and provides proper back support. If your mattress is not firm enough, have someone place a ½-inch-thick piece of plywood board between the mattress and box spring. Shop for specially made bed boards.

- Many mattresses are firm underneath but have a soft "pillow-top" covering that offers body support, but still has a cushiony feeling. Ask your doctor or physical therapist to recommend an appropriate mattress for your needs.

- Sleep with only one pillow under your head. Using two pillows may raise your head too much and cause neck pain.

- When purchasing a mattress, take the time to discuss the benefits of various mattresses with the salesperson. Ask to see any research material comparing various models.

- Lie down on various mattresses while you're shopping so you can see how they feel when you're in the sleeping position. Salespeople should encourage you to do so to be sure you are satisfied with your purchase.

- Don't try to go to sleep while still thinking about the stressful events of the day. Make sure you leave some time to read or clear your thoughts before going to sleep.

- Avoid caffeine later in the day. While a steaming cup of coffee might seem relaxing, caffeine is a stimulant that keeps you from falling asleep and sleeping soundly. Try an herbal, decaffeinated tea instead.

- If you like to sleep while lying on your stomach, be careful not to turn your neck too far toward your shoulder or to overarch your back. Place a pillow under your head to help keep it turned forward, minimizing neck rotation. Put another pillow under your stomach to flatten out any arch in your back.

- Don't drink tea, water or any liquid too close to your bedtime. Drinking close to bedtime may cause you to have to get out of bed to urinate during the night. You may find it difficult to go back to sleep.

- Regular, moderate exercise can keep your joints and muscles healthy, contributing to better sleeping, but don't exercise right before bedtime. Exercise causes your heart rate to accelerate and revs up the body, making it difficult to relax and go right to sleep.

- Establish a regular sleeping schedule. Your body will be better rested and function better if you are not sleeping late one day and forcing yourself to get up very early the next morning. It's important to stick to a regular bedtime and waking time, even on weekends.

- If you feel you must sleep with your upper body raised, place blocks or a board underneath the legs of the top of the bed. An adjustable bed also may be useful for you.

- Try not to sleep with a pillow underneath your knees, unless you are experiencing severe pain.

- If you like to sleep while lying on your back, sleep with a small rolled towel in your pillowcase or use a cervical or neck pillow to avoid stressing your neck or neck muscles.

- If you like to sleep while lying on your side, support your arms and legs with several soft pillows or a large body pillow.

Relaxing Before Bedtime

- A warm bath can be a great place to relax. Make time for your daily soak, whether in the morning to loosen stiff joints before your day, or in the evening to relax you before you sleep or have sex.

- Use caution when getting in or out of the bathtub. Use a sliding board to slide in, or install handrails to help you lower yourself in and raise yourself out of the tub. See Chapter Four for more specific techniques for safely using your bathtub.

- Don't use bath oils in your bath water. Oils make the bottom of the bathtub dangerously slippery, and may leave a film that will require extra effort to scrub clean.

- When leaning your head back in a bathtub, use a bath pillow to cushion the neck and support your head.

- Use a bath rack, a long plastic tray that fits across the bathtub, to hold soap, sponges and other items while you soak.

- Don't use candles around your bathtub. Candles can slip and fall onto bath rugs, causing a fire hazard. In addition, glass candle holders may fall into your bathtub and break, possibly causing cuts, slips or falls.

- If you can, make time each day for relaxation. Make it a formal event in your day, whether you are at home or at your workplace. Pick a quiet place and time of day when you won't be disturbed for at least 15 minutes. Make yourself as comfortable as possible before beginning. Loosen any tight clothing and uncross your legs, ankles and arms. Sit in a comfortable chair or lie down. Breathe slowly to release stress and relax your mind and body.

* If you wear a robe when you relax before bedtime, make sure it's not too long. Robe hems should reach no lower than the ankle to help prevent trips and falls.

* Alcoholic beverages may seem to relax you, but alcohol actually is a stimulant that will keep you from restful sleep. Drink only in moderation. If you are taking such medications as acetaminophen, discuss the possible dangers of drinking with your physician.

* Reading a good book can be a great way to relax. If you have difficulty holding a book, use a book stand.

* Prop up a book on a bed tray while you sit in bed, or use a lap desk with a hard surface and a cushioned bottom.

* Relaxation is an important component of self-management. Relaxation techniques such as yoga, water exercise, deep breathing or

just watching your favorite video may help you ease pain, decrease stress and fatigue, and go to sleep. Not all techniques work for everyone. If any relaxation techniques you try don't work, are unpleasant or increase your anxiety, find another way to relax.

× Try audio books if you can't hold up a regular book. Sit in a comfortable chair and listen to the book being read on your home stereo or tape deck.

× Music may help you relax and get to sleep. Use a clock radio that has a music timer. These radios can shut off after 30 minutes, so you can lull yourself to sleep with your favorite tunes.

× Sex is an important mode of relaxation for many people, and it is an important part of many relationships. Some sexual positions may be easier than others for people with arthritis. For a thorough guide to sex with arthritis, call 800/568-4045 and request a copy of the Arthritis Foundation's free publication A *Guide to Intimacy With Arthritis*. You should discuss your needs with your partner, and consult your health-care professional if you have concerns or questions.

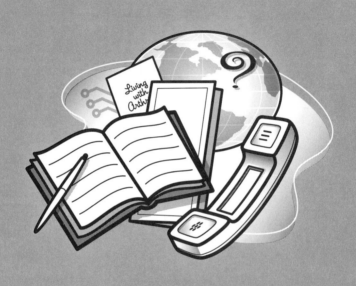

Resources *for* Good Living

T he mission of the Arthritis Foundation is to improve lives through leadership in the prevention, control and cure of arthritis and related diseases.

As a nonprofit organization, the Arthritis Foundation relies on your contributions to fund research, programs and services. You can make a difference in people's lives by becoming a member of the Arthritis Foundation. Please contact your local chapter or call **800/283-7800**. You will receive materials about the benefits of Arthritis Foundation membership, including the award-winning bimonthly magazine *Arthritis Today*. Log on to the Foundation Web site, **www.arthritis.org**, for more information about arthritis, Arthritis Foundation resources or to find the chapter nearest you.

Programs and Services

Most Arthritis Foundation chapters can provide a list of doctors in your area who specialize in the evaluation and treatment of arthritis and arthritis-related diseases.

EXERCISE PROGRAMS

The Arthritis Foundation sponsors, develops and coordinates exercise programs for people with arthritis, featuring specially trained instructors. These programs include:

- **Walk With Ease:** This course, accompanied by a book, shows you ways to develop a walking routine for fitness.
- **Arthritis Foundation Exercise Program:** These courses feature gentle movements to increase joint flexibility, range of motion, stamina and muscle strength. An accompanying video is available for home use. Call 800/283-7800 to order yours.
- **Arthritis Foundation Aquatic Program:** These water exercise programs help relieve strain on muscles and joints. An accompanying aquatic exercise video is available for home use. Call 800/283-7800 to order yours.

EDUCATIONAL AND SUPPORT GROUPS

The Arthritis Foundation sponsors mutual-support groups that provide opportunities for discussion and problem-solving among people with arthritis. In addition, the Arthritis Foundation offers the Arthritis Foundation Self-Help Program, which is designed to help people actively manage their particular disease through exercise, medications, relaxation techniques, pain management, nutrition and more.

Information and Products

Find the latest information about arthritis, including research, medications, government advocacy, programs and services, through one of the many information resources offered by the Arthritis Foundation:

WWW.ARTHRITIS.ORG

Information about arthritis is available 24 hours a day on the Internet at the Arthritis Foundation's interactive, comprehensive Web site. Find news about arthritis, ways to get involved, and a variety of useful arthritis products, including books, brochures, videos and more.

ARTHRITIS ANSWERS

Call toll-free at **800/283**-7800 for 24-hour, automated information about arthritis and Arthritis Foundation resources. Trained volunteers and staff also are available at your local Arthritis Foundation chapter to answer questions or refer you to physicians and other resources. For general questions about arthritis, you also can e-mail questions to **help@arthritis.org**.

PUBLICATIONS

The Arthritis Foundation offers many publications to educate people with arthritis, as well as their families and friends, about diagnosis, medications, exercise, diet, pain management and more.

- **Books** - The Arthritis Foundation publishes a variety of books on arthritis to help you understand and manage your condition, live a healthier life, and cope with the emotional challenges that come with a chronic illness. Order books directly at **www.arthritis.org**, or by calling **800/283-7800**. All Arthritis Foundation books are available in retail bookstores.

- **Brochures** - The Arthritis Foundation offers brochures containing concise, understandable information on the many arthritis-related diseases and conditions. Topics include surgery, the latest medications, guidance for working with your doctors, and self-managing your illness. Single copies are available free of charge at www.arthritis.org, or by calling **800/283-7800**.

× *Arthritis Today* - This award-winning, bimonthly magazine provides interesting feature articles in each issue, providing the latest information on research, new treatments, trends and tips from experts and readers to help you manage arthritis. Subscriptions are available for $12 per year, or you can get a one-year subscription to *Arthritis Today* as a benefit when you become a member of the Arthritis Foundation. Annual membership is $20 and helps fund research to find cures for arthritis. Call **800/283-7800** for information.

× *Kids Get Arthritis Too* - This newsletter, focusing on juvenile rheumatic diseases, is published six times a year. Features speak to children and teens with the illness, as well as to their parents. Stories examine the latest news in diagnosis, treatment and research of children's rheumatic diseases, as well as helpful ways kids can cope with their illnesses and the challenges they bring. This newsletter is available free to members of the Arthritis Foundation. Call **800/283-7800** or e-mail kgatmail@arthritis.org to sign up.

RESOURCES

The companies listed below are manufacturers of ergonomic office equipment and daily living equipment. You may request catalogs and purchase directly from the company or through your physical therapist, occupational therapist or health-care provider.

This list is by no means complete, but it gives you a good place to begin searching for useful products. Consult a physical or occupational therapist, or speak to your doctor to find more sources of self-help or assistive devices.

There also is a non-profit organization called Illinois Assistive Technology Project that helps people find assistive devices and maintains lists of companies that sell them. This organization can provide information specific to your state.

Illinois Assistive Technology Project
  1 West Old State Capitol Plaza
  Suite 100
  Springfield, IL 62701
  800/852-5110 (Illinois only)
  217/522-7985
  www.iltech.org

Daily Living Equipment
Aids For Arthritis, Inc.
  35 Wakefield Drive
  Medford, NJ 08055
  800/654-0707
  www.aidsforarthritis.com

Assistive Devices, Inc.
(ADI)
4000 Brandi Court
Austin, TX 78759-8109
800/856-0889
512/346-0889
www.assisteddevicesinc.com

Concepts ADL
10804 Mark Twain Road
West Frankfort, IL 62896
800/626-3153
www.adlrehab.com

Northcoast Medical Incorporated
18305 Sutter Boulevard
Morgan Hill, CA 95037
800/235-7054
www.beabletodo.com

Sears Health and Wellness Catalog
7700 Brush Hill Road
Burr Ridge, IL 60527
800/326-1750
www.searshealthandwellness.com

Sammons Preston Rolyan
Patterson Medical Company
P.O. Box 5071
Bolingbrook, IL 60440
800/558-8633
www.sammonspreston.com

Ergonomic Office Equipment
Ergo Source
4250 Norex Drive
Chaska, MN 55318-4374
800/969-4374

ErgoDirect
19 Newport Avenue
Selden, NY 11784
866/374-6347
www.ergodirect.net

Infogrip
1794 East Main Street
Ventura, CA 93001
805/652-0770
800/397-0921
info@infogrip.com